D0150439

THE HARVARD UNIVERSITY PRESS FAMILY HEALTH GUIDES

This book is meant to educate, but it should not be used as a substitute for personal medical advice. Readers should consult their physicians for specific information concerning their individual medical conditions. The authors have done their best to ensure that the information presented here is accurate up to the time of publication. However, as research and development are ongoing, it is possible that new findings will supersede some of the data presented here.

This book contains references to actual cases that Dr. Alpert has encountered. However, names and other identifying characteristics have been changed to protect the privacy of those involved.

Many of the designations used by manufacturers and sellers to distinguish their products are claimed as trademarks. Where those designations appear in this book and Harvard University Press was aware of a trademark claim, then the designations have been printed in initial capital letters (for example, Tylenol).

Spinal Cord Injury and the Family

A NEW GUIDE

Michelle J. Alpert, M.D.
Saul Wisnia

HARVARD UNIVERSITY PRESS
Cambridge, Massachusetts
London, England
2008

Illustrations by Arleen Frasca

Library of Congress Cataloging-in-Publication Data
Alpert, Michelle J., 1966–
    Spinal cord injury and the family : a new guide / Michelle J. Alpert,
Saul Wisnia.
        p.   cm.
    Includes bibliographical references and index.
    ISBN-13: 978-0-674-02714-5 (cloth : alk. paper)
    ISBN-10: 0-674-02714-0 (cloth : alk. paper)
    ISBN-13: 978-0-674-02715-2 (pbk. : alk. paper)
    ISBN-10: 0-674-02715-9 (pbk. : alk. paper)
    1. Spinal cord—Wounds and injuries—Popular works.   2. Spinal
cord—Wounds and injuries—Patients—Family relationships. I. Wisnia,
Saul. II. Title.
    RD594.3.A47   2008
    617.4′82044—dc22   2007050307

To Agi and Ed Alpert, who have been with me each step of the way, and I know always will be.

—MJA

To all the people with whom we talked while writing this book; their stories of challenge and fulfillment have been an inspiration.

—SW

Contents

Foreword by Cindy and Ted Purcell ... *ix*

Abbreviations ... *xiii*

1 Introduction to Spinal Cord Injury ... *1*

2 Early Days: The ER, Rehab, and Beyond ... *22*

3 Adjusting to SCI: The Return Home ... *53*

4 Back to Productivity: Work, School, and Play ... *73*

5 Dating after SCI: Out and About ... *110*

6 Sexual Function after SCI: The Next Challenge ... *123*

7 Couples and Relationship Issues: Making It Work ... *147*

8 Fertility and Pregnancy: The Possibilities ... *173*

9 Parenting with SCI: Moms and Dads on Wheels ... *200*

10 Children and Adolescents with SCI:

The Next Generation ... *236*

11 Medical Complications of SCI: Do's and Don'ts ... *265*

Appendix: Spinal Cord Injury by the Numbers ... *299*

Resources ... *303*

Suggested Reading ... *315*

Acknowledgments ... *327*

Index ... *331*

Foreword

We have led charmed lives. We've traveled all over the country, own a nice home in the suburbs, have full-time jobs, and are raising a happy, well-adjusted son who has many friends, plays sports, and loves to ride a dirt bike. One of us has fly-fished in exotic locations all over the world, and the other lectures to students and staff at colleges, universities, and corporations throughout our state. We coach our son's Little League team and are active volunteers in our hometown. We do all these things, yet we also both use wheelchairs as a result of spinal cord injuries. How can two people lead charmed lives from wheelchairs, you might ask? It's simple—not easy, but simple. We do it the same way anybody else does, but differently.

Spinal cord injury, or SCI, is a traumatic, life-altering experience that affects not only the individual suffering the injury but his or her family and friends as well. SCI is no less traumatic today than it was in the 1970s, when we were both injured, but healthcare and technology have changed, making the prospects of returning to a meaningful, productive life post-injury greater than ever. In the 1970s, people who had experienced injuries were just starting to look forward to brighter futures: a return to independence rather than interminable years spent in nursing homes or other long-term care facilities. Young soldiers injured in Vietnam, men and women hurt in automobile and diving accidents, and those paralyzed through other means were not satisfied sitting in sterile hospital rooms looking out at the world passing by them. So they went out and created opportunities for themselves.

In those early days, community resources were limited and much of the practical information needed to survive independently outside the hospital was available only through an informal peer network of individuals who had already "made it." At the rehab unit, when they showed you how to do things like change a catheter, they had all the supplies and equipment right there. When you went home, you didn't know where to get all the necessary medical supplies or even an inner tube for a wheelchair tire. You didn't know how to handle all the insurance questions you had, or how to hire personal care attendants—or PCAs, as we quickly learned they were called. If you asked the pharmacist at CVS where the "chux" were, he didn't know what you were talking about, but he could point you toward the disposable underpads.

More than once, our network of fellow SCI folks saved us. For every question, someone had the answer or could point us in the right direction: "You have to speak with Charlie, he's put hand controls in and out of his car several times; he can show you how to do it." "Call Ralph at such and such a pharmacy, they can get the catheters and leg bags you'll need." "Have you applied for Medicaid and been referred to vocational rehabilitation services?"

Today this type of network remains essential for a family struggling to adjust to life after spinal cord injury. Families often lose their identity and fall apart because so much energy is focused on helping the individual who is paralyzed. We saw many families grow apart as the stress of caring for a loved one and the changes it created in families' lives became overwhelming. Today families have access to many more resources—like this book—to help with daily life and the practical and emotional consequences that SCI brings. No one has to face spinal cord injury alone.

Twenty years ago when we told family and friends that we were planning to get married, many of them thought we were making a mistake. The reactions were similar seven years later when we decided to have a child. It wasn't that they believed our love wasn't sincere or that we wouldn't be good parents; it was just that they didn't think we could meet the challenges of these major life steps from the chairs where we spent so much of our days.

Their hearts were in the right place, but they were wrong. SCI does not need to be a barrier to having a happy home life and family. Not so long ago it did, and without proper resources and a strong social network, it can still have that effect. But for those armed with the ability to rebound from setbacks and stay focused on long-term goals, returning to a meaningful, productive, and fulfilling life is an attainable ambition. Doing so will take a partnership, with healthcare providers and rehab specialists, with friends, family, and community organizers. But we, and many like us, are living proof that this goal can be reached.

Spinal Cord Injury and the Family offers a comprehensive overview of how SCI affects the individual as well that person's family and friends. It also provides the most current information to those impacted by SCI, along with lots of practical advice for managing the many daily challenges as well as the less common ones. Armed with the information in this book, individuals and families will be able to focus on learning what they will need to recover from the trauma of paralysis and return to lives that, while surely different, can be as fulfilling as they were before.

Just ask our son, Tanner. In response to the question, "What's it like having two parents with SCI?" he said, "Sometimes it's hard because they can't come dirt biking and some other things with me, but sometimes it's fun because I get to go riding on their wheelchairs. It's good because I can still do everything other kids can do—and more."

We wish this book had been available when we were first injured. You can read it cover to cover or just focus on the chapters that pertain to you. In going through it, we were reminded of some of the challenges we've overcome. People with chronic illnesses like spinal cord injury have to tackle many difficult tasks every day, but these eventually become a part of their routine. Some people might look at you and say, "Wow, I'm glad I don't have to take ten minutes instead of thirty seconds to get in and out my car," but knowing this is the case, you learn to allow for the extra time and factor it into your day. To someone newly injured, or their friends and family members, these little things may seem monumental. For those who find themselves faced with them, this book has a lot to offer.

Yesterday Ted was fly-fishing for false albacore, bluefish, and striped bass while bouncing in the waves off Fishers Island in Long Island Sound. As he drifted by another boat, someone called out, "It's good to see a man with wheels out on the water." To us, that's just what Ted does. Ten years ago he had to convince the owner of a charter business that taking somebody in a wheelchair out on his boat was a good idea; now that man can advertise that his business is "wheelchair accessible." Tonight we're going out to dinner in the city, then to the theater. Our son is seeing a movie with friends. We're not sitting still, and neither should you. Read for yourselves.

Cindy and Ted Purcell

Abbreviations

AD	Autonomic dysreflexia
ADA	Americans with Disabilities Act
ADL	Activities of daily living
AHRQ	Agency for Healthcare Research and Quality (formerly the Agency for Health Care Policy and Research)
ART	Assisted reproductive technologies
BFO	Balanced forearm orthosis
CARF	Commission on Accreditation of Rehabilitation Facilities
CT	Computerized tomography
DVT	Deep venous thrombosis
ED	Erectile dysfunction
ER	Emergency room
FDA	Food and Drug Administration
GED	General Educational Development Diploma
ICU	Intensive care unit
ILC	Independent living center
IPE	Individual plan of employment
IPSA	International Professional Surrogate Association
IUD	Intrauterine device
IUI	Intrauterine insemination
IVF	In vitro fertilization
MRC	Massachusetts Rehabilitation Commission
MRI	Magnetic resonance imaging
NSCIA	National Spinal Cord Injury Association
NWBA	National Wheelchair Basketball Association
OT	Occupational therapist
PCA	Personal care attendant

PE	Pulmonary embolism
PM & R	Physical medicine and rehabilitation
PT	Physical therapist
SCI	Spinal cord injury
SSA	Social Security Administration
SSDI	Social Security Disability Insurance
SSI	Supplemental Security Income
TENS	Transcutaneous electrical nerve stimulation
UTI	Urinary tract infection
VAC	Vacuum-assisted closure
VRC	Vocational rehabilitation counselor
WOW	Winners on Wheels

SPINAL CORD INJURY AND THE FAMILY

Introduction to Spinal Cord Injury

I am not paralyzed, but I easily could have been. On the last day of my freshman year of college, I was hit by a car while crossing a street on campus. I don't remember any details of the accident, but after waking up in the hospital seven days later, I learned that I had been thrown from the car's hood and had sustained extensive orthopedic injuries. Although I had always wanted to be a doctor and had spent many hours volunteering at my hometown hospital as a teenager, up to that point I knew little about the rehabilitation process. Then I experienced it myself.

For the first time, while undergoing outpatient rehab over the next several months, I was directly exposed to people with significant physical disabilities. I often found it difficult to focus on my own physical and occupational therapy sessions because my attention was drawn to other patients nearby, many of whom were learning to maneuver their new wheelchairs or eat with specialized forks and knives. Several of these patients had spinal cord injuries, and while their situations were much more serious than my own—I *knew* I would walk again—they appeared anything but discouraged. They seemed to possess a fierce determination to move past the limitations of their "new" bodies with a resiliency I found inspiring.

Equally powerful were the relationships these individuals shared with their therapists. Strangers a short time before, caregivers and patients were now inexplicably linked by a resolve to tackle head-on the frustrations and joys of rehab. No matter how difficult a task or how slow the progress, they kept at it again and again. The dedication and intensely human connection between them made a deep and lasting impression on me. Unknowingly, during those long summer months, I was getting my first exposure to what would become my future career.

Shortly after returning to my pre-med courses a few months after my accident, I began volunteering on the pediatric rehab unit of C. S. Mott Children's Hospital, part of the University of Michigan Medical Center. Seven years later, when it came time to choose an area of concentration for my residency, I knew I wanted to be part of that world I had first seen from the inside. There could be no better way, I felt, to put my still-developing medical skills to work than to partner with therapists and other caregivers in an attempt to help people with disabilities resume their lives after injury. Today, when I receive a long letter from a patient who has recently gotten married or a card that reads simply, "Thanks for getting me back on my feet," I know I made the right decision.

Spinal cord injuries can happen to anyone—young or old, male or female, of any race, religion, or socioeconomic status. They are often caused by motor vehicle or diving accidents, but they can also result from medical conditions such as tumors or infections, gunshot wounds, falls, or freak accidents. In more than fifteen years of caring for individuals with spinal cord injury (SCI), I have encountered just about every possible scenario that can lead to this condition. By sharing some of my experiences and relying on the voices and stories of my patients, I hope to help readers more fully understand that people with SCI and their families can continue to live meaningful lives filled with personal, social, and vocational accomplishments. My husband, Saul Wisnia, a writer and author with a decade of experience covering the healthcare industry and an equal span as the spouse of a rehab doctor, was the logical choice to help me bring their stories and my experiences to print.

The first thing that people faced with spinal cord injury should realize is that they are far from alone. Each year in the United States, approximately 40 people per 1 million sustain traumatic spinal cord injuries, not including those who die at the scene of accidents. This translates into about 11,000 new traumatic injuries annually. (For a complete breakdown of SCI statistics, see the appendix.) Depending on the location of an SCI, movement and sensation may be lost in both the arms and the legs (tetraplegia, formerly known as quadriplegia), or just in the legs (paraplegia). Although most people assume that no one with tetraplegia can move or feel any part of their upper extremities, that's not the case: many people can actually still move some muscles of their arms, like their elbows, wrists, or a few fingers. Similarly, some individuals with paraplegia have enough remaining leg strength that they can walk with braces and crutches. Yet with the most extreme injuries, there is *no* movement of any extremity, and the person may even need a respirator to breathe.

No matter what their degree of function, life is far from over for those who have experienced spinal cord injury. An individual who experiences this trauma is still somebody's son or daughter, mother or father, friend or lover, colleague or coworker. Paralysis does not take away these special relationships or roles, but it can change them and add numerous challenges to a person's day-to-day existence. Through my own interactions with hundreds of SCI patients, I have found that those who are able to get past the initial negativity, educate themselves about their injury, and investigate the available resources are the ones most likely to adapt well to their new circumstances. By figuring out how to live with SCI and focus on what they *can* do rather than dwell on what they *can't,* they are able to maintain a strong and active presence within their families, communities, and society at large.

Family members and loved ones, too, find their lives altered as they indirectly face the changes brought on by SCI, whether that means assuming a new role as caregiver or having to find a new home without stairs. Getting to know patients and their families as they deal with the SCI experience together has given me a new appreciation for the human spirit and potential. By openly envisioning a future that may include a wheelchair, people who love and are committed to each other have succeeded by rearranging their lives in order to keep on living.

Basic Anatomy of the Spinal Cord

A complex and fragile bundle of nerve fibers bound like a cable and less than an inch wide, the spinal cord is the major connection between the brain and the rest of the body. It runs from the base of the brain down to the lower back and is surrounded by bone for protection. The spine (or vertebral column) serving as its shield is made up of a stack of twenty-nine individual bones (vertebrae) attached by ligaments and muscles. In between each pair lies a cushionlike tissue, the intervertebral disc, which acts as a shock absorber and protects the spine from the impact of regular human movement.

The spine is separated into four sections (see Figure 1). The top portion, the cervical segment, consists of seven vertebrae (commonly identified as C1-C7) that constitute the neck. Next down is the thoracic segment, twelve vertebrae (T1-T12) that run to the waist and attach to the ribs. The lower spine, or lumbar segment, has five vertebrae (L1-L5) and essentially constitutes the lower back. Lastly, there is the sacrum, or sacral segment, consisting of five fused vertebrae near the buttocks and above the tailbone (see Figure 2).

Inside this bony column runs the spinal cord, which transmits messages to the brain about different sensations—like temperature, position, and touch—and receives information back regarding movements of the arms, trunk (or torso), and legs.

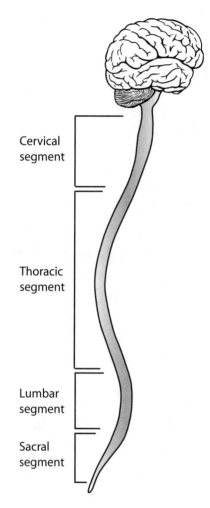

Cervical segment

Thoracic segment

Lumbar segment

Sacral segment

FIGURE 1.   The four sections of the spinal cord.

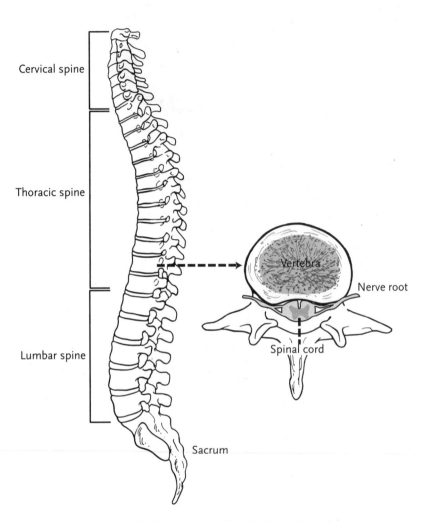

Cervical spine

Thoracic spine

Lumbar spine

Sacrum

Vertebra

Nerve root

Spinal cord

FIGURE 2.   The vertebral column (at left), which consists of twenty-nine stacked bones, or vertebrae. Like the spinal cord, the column is divided into four sections, including the sacrum. At right is a cross-section of a vertebra illustrating how the spinal cord runs through a tunnel provided by the stacked backbones.

Both of these message relays occur in a matter of milliseconds. For example, when someone pets a cat, sensory receptors in the person's hand send signals along nerves to her spinal cord and up to her brain. The sensation is then interpreted and experienced as soft and furry. By contrast, when a person is driving and a cat darts in front of his car, the brain analyzes this event as an emergency and relays a message through the driver's spinal cord to move his foot and slam on the brakes.

The spinal cord ends at the level of the first or second lumbar vertebrae, and, like the bony spine, it is divided into four sections: cervical, thoracic, and lumbar. Each is responsible for controlling a particular part of the body. Specifically, the cervical spinal cord carries information related to movement and feeling to and from the upper body, arms, and hands; the thoracic cord does the same for the trunk; and the lumbar cord, for the lower body and legs. In all three sections, the sensory information and the motor information travel through different pathways, so that someone might be able to feel his leg even if he can't move it. After the last section of the spinal cord (L1 or L2), a group of loosely bound nerves known as the lower lumbar and sacral cord continues downward. These nerves are referred to as the *cauda equina* (Latin for horse's tail), and they are responsible for controlling bowel, bladder, and sexual functions, as well as the motor and sensory control of some leg muscles.

With an injury to the spinal cord, the messaging system between the brain and particular parts of the body breaks down. Critical information about the body's sensation can no longer be interpreted by the brain, which, in turn, cannot relay its movement signals to specific muscles. This damage can be caused by the impact resulting from automobile accidents, by falls, gunshot wounds, and other traumatic events, or by medical problems such as strokes, tumors, infections, or conditions that disrupt the blood supply to the spinal cord.

Trauma to the spinal cord usually causes significant shifting of the vertebrae, which then pinch or crush the spinal cord within. This is what typically results when bones in the back are broken or ligaments are torn in a car crash. Torn fragments of bone or disc may then enter the bony canal where the spinal cord sits and also directly injure—by bruising, tearing, or cutting—its nervous tissue. In other cases, such as falls, the spinal cord may only be bruised and no bones broken, yet the resultant swelling is enough to seriously damage the tissue. Trauma-induced bleeding into the spinal cord, such as may occur with stab wounds, is yet another way that the cord's message-carrying ability can be disrupted.

Levels of Injury

No matter what causes spinal cord damage, the injured person will experience changes in movement, sensation, bladder control, and other bodily functions (see Table 1). The parts of the body affected depend on the section of the spinal cord involved. In the most general terms, the higher up in the cord (toward the neck) an injury occurs, the more parts of the body may be paralyzed—and, subsequently, the greater the potential loss of function. In describing the injury and resulting patterns of weakness and sensory loss, physicians and other medical professionals use letters and numbers that refer to the section and level of spinal cord involved (for example, C7 or L2).

Tetraplegia

Serious injury to the neck or top of the spinal cord (the cervical area) can result in tetraplegia. This type of injury can happen numerous ways, usually in a single moment.

While attending a party, Pablo was out on the balcony with some friends. Suddenly, the deck collapsed, sending the group crashing

Table 1. Functional outcomes for patients with complete SCI

Level of injury	A.M. care	Feeding	Grooming	Dressing
C3, C4	Total dependence	May be unable to feed self. Use of BFOs with universal cuff and adapted utensils indicated; drinks with long straw after set up	Total dependence	Total dependence
C5	Independent with specially adapted devices after set up	Independent with specially adapted equipment for feeding after set up	Independent with specially adapted equipment for grooming after set up	Assistance with upper-extremity dressing; dependent for lower-extremity dressing
C6	Independent with equipment	Independent with equipment; drinks from glass	Independent with equipment	Independent with upper-extremity dressing; assistance needed for lower-extremity dressing
C7	Independent	Independent	Independent with equipment	Potential for independence in upper- and lower-extremity dressing with equipment
C8, T1	Independent	Independent	Independent	Independent
T2–T10	Independent	Independent	Independent	Independent
T11–L2	Independent	Independent	Independent	Independent
L3–S3	Independent	Independent	Independent	Independent

Table 1. Functional outcomes for patients with complete SCI *(continued)*

Level of injury	Bathing	Bowel and bladder routine	Bed mobility	Pressure relief
C3, C4	Total dependence	Total dependence	Total dependence	Independent in powered recliner wheelchair; dependent in bed or manual wheelchair
C5	Total dependence	Total dependence	Needs assistance of other and equipment	Most require assistance
C6	Independent in upper- and lower-extremity bathing with equipment	Independent for bowel routine; assistance needed with bladder routine	Independent with equipment	Independent
C7	Independent with equipment	Independent	Independent	Independent
C8, T1	Independent	Independent	Independent	Independent
T2–T10	Independent	Independent	Independent	Independent
T11–L2	Independent	Independent	Independent	Independent
L3–S3	Independent	Independent	Independent	Independent

Table 1. Functional outcomes for patients with complete SCI *(continued)*

Level of injury	Wheelchair transfers	Wheelchair propulsion	Ambulation	Transportation
C3, C4	Total dependence	Independent in pneumatic or chin-control–driven power wheelchair with powered reclining feature	Not applicable	Dependent on others in accessible van with lift; unable to drive
C5	Assistance of one person with or without transfer board	Independent in powered chair indoors and outdoors; short distances in manual wheelchair with lugs indoors	Not applicable	As above
C6	Potentially independent with transfer board	Independent in manual wheelchair with plastic rims or lugs indoors; assistance needed outdoors and with elevators	Not applicable	Independent driving in specially adapted van
C7	Independent with or without transfer board including car, except to/from floor with assistance	Independent in manual wheelchair indoors and outdoors, except curbs, stairs	Not applicable	Independent driving in car with hand controls or specially adapted van; independent wheelchair-into-car placement
C8, T1	Independent including to/from floor and car	Independent in manual wheelchair indoors and outdoors; curbs, escalators	Not applicable	As above
T2–T10	Independent	Independent	Exercise only (not functional with orthoses): requires physical assistance or guarding	As above
T11–L2	Independent	Independent	Potential for independent functional ambulation indoors with orthoses: some have potential for stairs using railing	As above
L3–S3	Independent	Independent	Community ambulation: independent indoors and outdoors with orthoses	As above

Source: Joel DeLisa et al., *Rehabilitation Medicine: Principles and Practice,* 2nd ed. (Philadelphia: Lippincott, 1993).

twenty feet to the ground below. Pablo's fourth cervical vertebra was broken (C4), damaging his spinal cord at that level and paralyzing him from the neck down. Although he initially needed a ventilator, Pablo was eventually able to breathe on his own because the diaphragm—the primary muscle responsible for breathing—receives most of its messages from a part of the spinal cord located above the injured area. He still possessed head and neck control, so he learned to propel his new electric wheelchair with a "sip and puff" mechanism and to operate a computer by using a stick held in his mouth. But because his SCI left him without the use of his arms (beyond shoulder shrugs) and his legs, Pablo needed help with his personal care, including bathing, dressing, and eating.

"My life had changed, but I got through rehab and was able to go on to law school," Pablo recalls. "I was lucky I had a personal care attendant [PCA] to take notes for me in class and help me with other daily tasks like bathing, dressing in the morning, and getting to bed at night. I'm proud of the fact that three years later I graduated, passed the bar, and became a practicing attorney. Paralysis didn't stop me."

Scott was shot in the neck at close range during a robbery at the convenience store where he worked. The bullet damaged his spinal cord at the sixth cervical level (C6), leaving his hands, chest, and lower body paralyzed. After months in rehabilitation, the nineteen-year-old could manage some of his own activities of daily living (or ADLs), but he needed an attendant for most of his lower body care. He learned to use adaptive equipment like plate guards (to prevent food from falling off dishes), long-handled shoehorns, and a shower chair. When out in the community he needed a power wheelchair because of his decreased upper-body and arm strength, but he learned to propel a manual chair for exercise indoors.

"During rehab, I was lucky there were a couple of other kids my age there who had spinal cord injuries," Scott says. "We hung out

together, talked a lot, and pulled for each other while working out in the gym or learning how to get in and out of cars. Because those guys were so important to me in my recovery, I decided to help others going through the same thing by volunteering as a 'peer visitor' encouraging new rehab patients. I'm also thinking about going back to college for a degree in psychology."

Paraplegia

When the spinal cord is injured below the cervical segment, such as within the thoracic or lumbar area, the lower body and legs are affected, leaving the individual with the full use of his or her arms and hands. These people have paraplegia.

Martha, a physician, hated going to the doctor herself and usually just self-treated her own aches and pains. One day she developed gradually increasing mid-back discomfort that was not relieved with the usual over-the-counter medications. Reluctantly, she drove to her own hospital's emergency room, was evaluated by a colleague, and had X-rays taken. They looked normal, so she was sent home with stronger pain medications.

"Later that night, I developed a fever and my legs became weak," she remembers. "It got so bad I couldn't walk, so I went back to the hospital—this time by ambulance. I had an MRI [magnetic resonance imaging] taken of my spine, which showed an infection involving the lining of my spinal cord [at the fifth thoracic (T5) level]. By the time they started antibiotics, part of my lower chest and legs were numb and paralyzed."

Martha was an avid participant in her rehabilitation, and her physical and occupational therapists could barely keep up with her. "It was hard for me to be the patient rather than the doctor, so I wanted to get home as soon as possible," she recalls. "I worked as hard as I could to build up the strength in my arms, hoping my legs would eventually come back. Before my injury I couldn't even do one pushup, but only a month after, I could bench-press twenty pounds. By the time I was discharged to home I was able to dress and bathe myself. And when I went back to work a little while later, I did my rounds in a lightweight wheelchair. Needless to say, I have a newfound appreciation for what it's like to be a patient."

When the spinal cord is injured low enough (for example, at the lumbar level), the trunk and arms will be completely spared and only variable degrees of leg weakness or total paralysis will result in addition to bowel, bladder, and sexual dysfunction. For individuals with this type of injury, rehabilitation efforts are focused on strengthening the upper body and any preserved leg muscles, as well as learning to do self-care from a wheelchair. Depending on their remaining lower-body strength and how motivated they are, they may also be able to walk with braces and crutches. I have found that patients are usually very excited about the prospect of standing again. Even if they are not able to walk, the psychological benefits of standing upright are worth the effort. Standing exercises can also help with trunk control and overall reconditioning.

Andy was responsible for all the yard work and maintenance at his family's house. Each fall, he raked and disposed of the leaves, and once the trees were bare, he emptied the roof gutters of debris. One November day, he noticed that the gutters were overflowing with dead leaves and branches. Intending to do a quick cleanup, he set up his ladder and began climbing toward the roof. "I was moving too fast and lost my footing," he explains. "I fell to the ground and felt intense pain in my lower back. My legs wouldn't move, so I just tried to crawl inside and yelled for my wife."

Emergency room X-rays showed a fracture of the first lumbar vertebra. After undergoing surgery to realign and stabilize his spine,

Andy was transferred to a rehabilitation facility for a month, where he learned to walk short distances with long leg braces. Because this kind of walking required so much energy, however, he found himself using a wheelchair most of the time when he returned home. Independent in every other way, he even began driving with hand controls. "When I first realized I was paralyzed, I thought my life was over," he says. "Now that I'm able to do almost everything I could before, being in a wheelchair isn't nearly as big a deal as I thought it would be."

Since the spinal cord is shorter than the vertebral column and ends at the level of the first lumbar vertebra, an injury to the back will often affect only the very lower lumbar and/or sacral nerves (the *cauda equina*). A herniated lower lumbar disc or growing lumbrosacral tumor, for example, can compress the *cauda equina* that lies near it. Individuals with this level of injury may have weakness in just their feet or hips, requiring the use of short leg braces to support their ankles and keep their toes from dragging while walking. As with almost every other spinal cord injury, their bowel, bladder, and sexual systems are also affected, and learning various methods to manage these changes is usually one of the major focuses of rehabilitation.

Completeness of Injury

The severity of the damage to the spinal cord, in addition to its location, will dictate how much paralysis a person will experience. More specifically, spinal cord injuries are referred to as "complete" or "incomplete" depending on the extent of paralysis. With a complete injury, there is a total disruption of communication between the brain and the rest of the body at the level of damage; no messages can be relayed up or down the spinal cord below the point of injury, to or from the rest of the body, so *all*

voluntary movement and sensation beneath that level is eliminated. Many people assume that the cord must be severed for
someone to have such a catastrophic injury, but this degree of
paralysis can occur even with just a bruise to the cord. Complete
injuries will almost always result in some loss of sexual ability
and changes in bowel and bladder control.

With incomplete injuries, because the damage is only partial,
some exchange of information is still possible between the brain
and various body parts through the spinal cord. Subsequently,
some motor messages can still get past the area of damage to
the arms and legs, and some information about sensation can
travel up and be received and interpreted by the brain. Only partial loss of movement and sensation results below the injured
area. For example, an individual with incomplete tetraplegia will
have some weakness in all four limbs but will still be able to
move some muscles in his arms and/or even his legs. Time and
again, I have seen intensive inpatient occupational and physical
therapies, along with a person's determination and patience,
strengthen weak muscles—and in some cases bring about new
movement in muscles that had been completely paralyzed. Incomplete spinal cord injuries offer the best chance for recovery,
but how much function returns often depends upon the location
and extent of the damage.

*Mike had been having lower-back pain since a summer bicycle acci-
dent two years earlier. He had never seen a doctor for this problem
because it had never gotten bad enough to keep the thirty-year-old
electrician away from his job. One day, however, the pain became so
intense that he could barely stand upright. He noticed a "pins and
needle-like" feeling in his right leg, and he found it harder to pick his
feet up to walk. When he began to have trouble urinating, he decided it was time to go to the emergency room.*

"By then my entire right leg was paralyzed, and I couldn't move

the toes on my left foot," Mike recalls. "I had an MRI, and they found a spinal cord tumor. I wondered how long it had been there; the doctors couldn't tell me, and they thought it might have been the cause of my pain all along, not my bike crash." Mike was admitted to the hospital immediately. He underwent surgery to remove the growth and after a few days went on to rehabilitation. There his bladder function and some leg strength returned, and he eventually learned to walk with the help of a cane and a brace on his right leg.

People with incomplete injuries have different patterns of recovery. Sometimes, for instance, when only one side of the spinal cord is damaged, only one side of the body (the left or right) is weakened. In one type of incomplete tetraplegia called central cord syndrome, legs may recover more strength than arms. Individuals with this condition will usually be able to walk but may need help getting dressed. In many incomplete injuries, bowel and bladder function will eventually return to normal, and muscle strength can continue to improve for eighteen to twenty-four months after the incident. Furthermore, research has shown that the greater degree of strength regained shortly after injury (that is, within the first two months), the higher the likelihood that a person will have a strong long-term recovery and be able to walk again and/or use their arms.

Impact on the Family

Regardless of the extent of the damage, spinal cord injury is always a life-changing event, for the injured person as well as for his or her family and loved ones. When I notice that friends and family of my SCI patients are having a particularly hard time during the early days of hospitalization and rehab, I explain that it is often more difficult for those *watching* someone struggle to regain her life after paralysis than it is for the person herself. Patients are "in the trenches"; each day they awaken in the hospital with a clearly defined task ahead. Their time, especially during rehab, is regimented and goal-driven, with a full schedule of therapy sessions and community outings. Family members and loved ones, though they may be encouraged by the progress they see, must return home each night to reminders, both physical and emotional, that their son, mother, spouse, or lover will have a very different life once inpatient rehabilitation is over.

Yet despite all the changes, many families are, in fact, equipped to cope with the psychosocial issues that accompany a spinal cord injury. Members learn to reorganize their roles within the unit and to communicate openly with one another while also accepting support and assistance from friends, relatives, colleagues, and others. By sharing their feelings and fears, family members may actually grow closer during this time. Although each situation is different, the level to which new paralysis disrupts a family can depend as much on the group's coping skills and how it has managed crises in the past as on the severity of the injury itself.

Consider, for example, the spouse or partner of someone who has just experienced a spinal cord injury. If a paralyzed person can't return to his job, his significant other may have to make up the lost income. When the primary homemaker is injured, on the other hand, her partner may need to take on more domestic duties or hire extra help—which can affect both the family's finances and its privacy. While partners whose work lives were previously spent outside the home may have trouble adjusting to the changes, and perhaps even resent them, many couples are eventually able to rearrange their roles. Sex after SCI presents challenges of its own, but with a little creativity and determination, these too can be conquered.

An injured parent's paralysis presents a different set of obstacles. Although young children whose parents are going through a long hospitalization and rehab will miss the daily guidance they get from Mom or Dad, many will be able to manage the transition successfully if they are encouraged to take an active role in the process. Children can visit the hospital regularly and meet caregivers, join their parents for meals, and even attend therapy sessions. At the same time, however, children will need to adjust to changes in family dynamics as able-bodied parents or other adults assume more significant roles in their care. If the family moves to a more accessible home, children may have to switch schools. Although such a change can be tumultuous, it can also be regarded as a chance for children to make new friends and establish a new support system outside the home.

The parents of a child with spinal cord injury face their own set of challenges. Their son or daughter's day-to-day life will change dramatically, and along with it their own hopes and dreams. If an accident is the cause of the paralysis, they may blame themselves for not adequately protecting their child from danger; if one parent gave the child permission to do whatever caused the incident, he or she may feel guilt while the other parent feels anger. At the same time they are experiencing these emotions, other children in the family may need reassurance—both that their brother or sister will be okay and that their own needs will be met. Depending on how a family responds, these and other changes have the potential to either break down or strengthen it. Family members must now work together to get through the initial adjustment after an injury and reestablish new routines and rituals, while preserving as much of the past as possible.

As I've told families many times, a positive attitude is essential to adjusting to life after SCI. Some newly injured individuals become so angry over their physical changes that tension and anxiety fill their homes. Family members, frustrated by seemingly unreasonable demands for attention, may avoid helping out—a reaction that can magnify the injured person's feelings of loss. Siblings may feel forgotten or resent the extra time devoted to their injured brother or sister, while parents who overprotect their newly injured child may actually end up limiting their son's or daughter's independence and reducing his or her self-esteem.

Because spinal cord injury often forces family members to reconsider their roles within the unit, it may cause some initial resentment, though most people come to accept the situation. A stay-at-home mom who becomes paralyzed may initially feel a great sense of loss because she can no longer perform her household chores as before, but she can eventually learn ways to manage them from a wheelchair. Her husband, meanwhile, might grow to resent his new duties cleaning the kitchen and picking up the kids from soccer practice, until he realizes the stronger bonds he is forming with the children and his wife. A newly disabled teen may intentionally ignore his doctor's advice and develop dangerous complications such as bed sores in an attempt to "control" his parents and gain their attention; eventually, however, he may see the importance of a healthy lifestyle and the freedom, as well as the parental respect, that it brings. The key for families is to keep the lines of communication open and to accept one another's reactions as part of the healing process.

In the pages that follow, we explore the challenges faced by people with SCI and their families, and the many ways they successfully adapt after such a devastating occurrence. Chapters 2 and 3 look at paralyzed individuals as a group, focusing first on their initial hospitalization and rehabilitation, then on their return home. Chapter 4 examines the challenges and triumphs of adapting to disability and seeking the community resources necessary for a return to work, school, or other pursuits beyond one's front door. Chapters 5 through 7 delve into the complexities of interpersonal relationships—from dating to sexual exploration to committed unions—as well as the role changes and caregiver issues encountered by couples in which one or both members are paralyzed.

Next we address the joys and challenges faced by those who choose to conceive, bear, and raise children after paralysis: Chapter 8 focuses on fertility and pregnancy issues after injury, while Chapter 9 focuses on raising children without the full use of one's limbs. Chapter 10 deals with what parents can expect when the roles are reversed and a child is either injured or born with a spinal cord problem. The final chapter addresses the medical complications faced by even the strongest individuals in the years after an injury.

Although no two cases are exactly the same, the overriding message does not change: No matter what their support system or level of injury, people with SCI can adjust and move forward. No doubt they will experience significant lifestyle changes that will require patience and resolve. Family members and friends must work to understand these changes, as well as their own needs and feelings. Only through this kind of determination, healthy attitude, and proper knowledge can everybody come together to form the support system that is so crucial to tackling the daily challenges ahead. I've seen it so many times in my work: By functioning as one and drawing on their collective strengths, disabled individuals and those who support them have learned to cope with their situations and regain full, meaningful lives. You can, too.

2

Early Days: The ER, Rehab, and Beyond

A few months after Matt turned forty, he took his family on a ski trip to Vermont as a birthday gift to himself. Looking back, he can still remember the details of what happened. "I went off a jump, and even though I didn't land it clean, I didn't fall. I wish I had. By the time I regained my balance I was about to hit a tree and couldn't stop. I never lost consciousness; I just fell to my knees and felt a zing in my back. I tried to move my toes, couldn't, and knew right away I was paralyzed."

Matt's wife and daughters, who had been skiing alongside him, rushed down to the lodge and came back with the ski patrol and a stretcher. Matt was transported by ambulance to a nearby hospital, where he was diagnosed with T10 paraplegia. Doctors performed emergency surgery in which rods were inserted into his back to support his broken spine. A week later, after Matt and his wife told their four young children that Daddy may never walk again, he was transferred to a large rehabilitation facility. There he learned the key to not feeling sorry for himself: keeping busy.

"There were about sixty of us there who were spinal cord injured," *Matt explains,* "and we had at least four sessions every day—physical therapy, occupational therapy, some type of classroom study, and awareness classes. They covered bowel movements, sexuality, getting back into the community, and reacting to different situations. There was a kitchen where we learned to move around, cook, and vacuum, and we spent a day at the airport learning how to check in,

get through crowds, and board a plane. We even took driving les-
sons. They just put us in a car with hand controls and said, 'Drive.'"

Reflecting on his days in rehab, Matt admits that he did worry
about whether he would still be able to be a good husband and fa-
ther despite being in a wheelchair. And even though his boss had
sent him a laptop so that Matt could stay connected to the office
during his hospitalization, he was skeptical about returning to his
job. Still, he remained determined not to wind up like the guys on
the unit who skipped therapy and spent most of the day in bed. "I
just felt like I couldn't afford to focus on the negative," Matt says. "I
was still alive, and that's what was important. I just wanted to get
home as quickly—and as strong—as I could."

Spinal cord injury irrevocably alters a person's life, introduc-
ing changes that are unanticipated, sudden, and (possibly) permanent. In an instant the future seems uncertain, and things
previously taken for granted now require thought and effort.
Just getting out of bed and preparing for the day becomes a major production. Emptying one's bowels and bladder is no longer
an ordinary, automatic process—now it takes a special routine
and can be a source of worry and potential embarrassment. The
once-simple task of dressing requires specialized equipment or
another person's help. All spontaneity seems to be gone, and going from one place to the next involves planning and preparation. Stairs may become a huge challenge, as can curbs on the
street. Even sex, though still possible, needs to be approached in
an entirely new way.

In short, little appears the way it was before. My patients
with SCI often speak of their lives as being divided into two
parts: before paralysis and after. They frequently view the past
with a kind of sadness, as the time when "things were normal"
or "before everything changed." The future, at least initially, can
be a blank and frightening slate for them. Many questions arise:

How will I earn a living? How will people react to me? Will I have to move to a new home? Will anybody find me attractive? What will sex be like? Why did this have to happen to me?

As I tell patients and their families, the key for people going through rehab is to move ahead. I certainly never mean to downplay the impact of SCI—it is always a devastating ordeal for everyone involved—but experience has shown me that patients rarely benefit from dwelling on the way life was pre-injury. Instead, they are better served focusing their energy on creating a *new* life and learning to work within the limitations of SCI. People need not abandon all their hopes and dreams because they are no longer as mobile as they once were, but they do need to realize that they now have a new starting point.

Initial Hospitalization

At the scene of an accident, fall, or other trauma, any individual suspected of having a spinal cord injury requires immediate medical attention. The preservation of life and protection of the spinal cord are the primary focus of emergency personnel. Neck collars and backboards are used to stabilize the spine and prevent any movement that might cause further damage to the spinal cord. People with certain injuries to the neck may also need help breathing. Rapid transfer to a trauma center, either by ambulance or by helicopter, is crucial. During this transport, the injured person usually receives intravenous steroids—the current standard of care for people with acute traumatic SCI.

Upon arrival at the hospital, the patient is brought to the emergency ward, where a team of physicians, nurses, and support staff begin a comprehensive but rapid medical assessment. Their first goal is to ensure that breathing and circulation are adequate, and then to determine the extent of neurological damage and the presence of any other serious injuries. X-rays and other imaging studies such as CT (computerized tomography) scans and MRIs are conducted to identify the specific fractures of the vertebral column, as well as any damage to the spinal cord and surrounding tissues. A careful neurological evaluation will determine the level of the spinal cord injury and the severity of the paralysis. This involves testing the strength of specific muscles as well as the sensation in the four extremities (arms and legs), torso (chest and abdomen), and rectal area.

After these initial tests, most patients will be transferred to the intensive care unit (ICU) for close monitoring. The majority will then go on to have some sort of surgical procedure within the first few days of admission. The purpose of these operations, which are performed by either an orthopedic surgeon or a neurosurgeon, is to relieve pressure on the spinal cord that may be caused by fractures, bone fragments, or bleeding, as well as to stabilize the spine with the help of metal plates and screws or bone grafts.

Within a couple of days after surgery, most patients are fit with some sort of support such as a back brace or collar in order to limit movement of the injured portion of the spine and to allow the bones and soft tissue to heal. These devices are usually worn whenever someone is up and out of bed. Some people with specific cervical spine injuries may instead be placed in a halo brace, a ring of metal that is attached to the head by small pins drilled into the skull, and then connected by rods to a plastic vest worn around the chest. This apparatus provides maximal stability to the cervical spine and, thereby, the spinal cord. The brace may be uncomfortable at first and cause some difficulty with swallowing (to be discussed later).

The good news is that these operations and braces make it possible for patients in the ICU to start sitting up and even getting out of bed without risk of further damage to the spinal cord. This is also the point at which rehabilitation should begin.

Some trauma centers have physicians on staff who specialize in physical medicine and rehabilitation (PM & R) and are available for consultation with the acute team. Early attention to rehabilitation concerns will help prevent future complications and enable patients to be mobilized as soon as possible. A PM & R physician like myself (also known as a physiatrist) may, for example, order specialized mattresses to prevent skin breakdown and ankle braces to maintain feet in the optimal position. In addition, this doctor may provide recommendations about bowel and bladder care.

In the acute care setting, the physiatrist also helps initiate and then coordinate the patient's rehabilitation plan with the physical therapists (PTs) and occupational therapists (OTs). Both PTs and OTs will conduct their own extensive evaluations of muscle strength and sensation as well as function. On the basis of their results, they will then design individualized exercise programs and treatment plans. At this point, prevention of joint contracture (a condition in which the joint becomes tight and difficult to move) is of utmost importance because the patient spends so much of his or her time prior to surgery immobilized. Once the surgeon determines that the patient may begin treatment, therapists will start range-of-motion exercises, passively moving the joints as much as possible to keep them flexible. Since these exercises are most beneficial when done several times a day, OTs and PTs frequently teach family members how to do them during their hospital visits. I have found that enabling loved ones to participate as caregivers early in the process provides them with an excellent opportunity to bond with the injured person both physically and emotionally. At the same time, it allows them to feel as though they are contributing to their loved one's care.

Physical and occupational therapists also have their own specific roles during the acute care phase. Depending on an individual's level of injury and other medical concerns, PTs may help with mobility tasks, including bed mobility, the process of turning from side-to-side and sitting up in bed; and transferring, moving from bed to wheelchair and back again. OTs also help with stretching and strengthening exercises, but primarily those involving the shoulders, elbows, and hands. In some cases, OTs may make hand splints to prevent discomfort and help keep a patient's fingers from becoming contracted. During this time, both OTs and PTs also begin to familiarize patients and family members with rehabilitation terms and techniques. In addition, speech and language pathologists may also initiate swallowing evaluations for those with cervical spinal cord injuries. (The further role of OTs, PTs, and speech therapists will be described in more detail below.)

On to Rehabilitation

"At rehab they were way more uplifting," Charlie remembers of his first days after transfer from acute care for C4-C5 tetraplegia. "I finally got to hear some positive things from the doctors and nurses. In the ICU, all I was hearing about was how I could never walk. At rehab, they thought I could get my arms back; they got me out of bed and started me on physical therapy. Because I'm good with my hands and like figuring out how things work, it took me about two minutes to get the hang of the 'sip-and-puff' wheelchair [a power chair controlled either by sucking in ("sipping") or by blowing out ("puffing") on a tube or straw held in the mouth]. I took it out for a spin around the hospital a couple times and was finally able to sit up and put my shoulders back. It was very uplifting, and it made me eager to work more on my hands. I knew I probably wasn't going to walk again, but now I was focusing on the things I could do."

Eventually, when an individual's acute medical condition has been stabilized, he or she is ready for the move to rehabilitation.

Many patients come to rehab directly from the intensive care unit, and the change can be dramatic. They now have access to doctors and other healthcare providers with time to explain carefully what has happened to them and what can be expected down the road. I have found that by speaking frankly and openly with patients and their families, and by affirming how stressful and even unreal this situation can be, I am able to help them understand more fully their specific needs and concerns—concerns that we can address together and on which the interdisciplinary team (see below) can focus when working with the patient during the weeks and months ahead.

In some cases, the move to rehabilitation involves transitioning to a rehab floor in the same hospital; in others, it means transferring to a separate, specialized rehabilitation facility. Insurance issues, personal choice, and bed availability are all factors that can determine where a person will receive rehabilitation. The level of injury may also play a role. Some hospitals, for instance, don't have the expertise to manage individuals who have tetraplegia and are ventilator-dependent, whereas other facilities may not have the equipment or staff to manage patients with tracheostomies (breathing tubes).

No matter where rehab takes place, the goal is the same. In contrast to acute care, where the focus is on saving life, rehab teaches patients how to *live* life. As a result, the level of patient participation increases dramatically. In the acute phase, patients spend most of their time in bed being cared for by others, but in rehab they are expected to participate as fully as possible in their daily regimen. Rehab is also the time when most people begin to realize the extent of their paralysis and the impact it will have on their lives. Because rehabilitation stays are measured in weeks rather than in days, patients have a chance to make progress and begin learning to live with their disability.

The goals of rehab are to prevent complications, maximize an individual's remaining abilities, and teach ways to compensate for new impairments. A major focus is education: teaching the person about his or her paralysis, as well as the techniques needed to get back to life and return home. If they are available, family members and significant others are encouraged to be an integral part of this training. For many newly injured patients, however, transfer to rehabilitation can be a mixed blessing. While it signifies survival, it also confirms that the patient has experienced a major, life-altering event and must learn to live with new physical limitations. Accordingly, many individuals often feel conflicted in the early days of rehab. Although they appear interested in learning more about spinal cord injury, their emotions may prevent them from fully grasping the information.

The Interdisciplinary Team

The interdisciplinary team plays an essential role in the patient's journey to functional recovery. A physician, most often a physiatrist like myself, coordinates the team, which usually consists of a rehabilitation nurse, physical therapist, occupational therapist, speech and language pathologist, case coordinator, psychologist, and therapeutic recreation specialist. In some cases, vocational rehabilitation specialists, dietitians, chaplains, and rehabilitation engineers may also join the team. The makeup of the group depends on the injured person's specific needs, as well as on the facility's resources.

Here is a quick look at some of the key individuals a patient is likely to encounter during a stay in rehab:

The *physiatrist* manages all the individual's medical care (sometimes in coordination with an internal medicine specialist), attempting to prevent any complications that may occur as a result of the SCI. He or she is responsible for leading interdisciplinary conferences at which the team meets to discuss each aspect of the patient's care and progress and to solve problems as they arise.

The *rehabilitation nurse* provides numerous services in addition to the usual nursing care. He or she works with the physician to manage skin care as well as to institute the patient's bowel and bladder programs. Many individuals with SCI are unable to empty their bladder and will need intermittent catheterization (a procedure in which a thin plastic tube is inserted several times daily into the bladder to drain urine and then removed). The rehab nurse is also responsible for teaching this technique to family members and patients who still have adequate hand function. Other patients will manage their bladder with an indwelling catheter, which remains in the bladder at all times, attached to a drainage bag to collect the urine. Nurses also instruct families on how to tend to the catheter, including how to change it monthly.

In addition, rehabilitation nurses work with patients to establish daily bowel programs that usually involve the use of suppositories at a specific time. This regular routine enables patients to have predictable bowel movements and avoid accidents. If patients have adequate trunk strength to transfer from their wheelchairs to a toilet or commode, occupational therapists will work with the nursing staff to determine the best and safest technique. This is just one example of how nurses and therapists collaborate to ensure that skills such as transfers learned by patients in the gym are carried over onto the hospital unit.

Just as in acute care, the primary role of the *physical therapist (PT)* continues to be enhancing skills needed for mobility, such as strength, balance, and flexibility. Once these basic goals are met, PTs can begin focusing on more functional activities like chair-to-car and bed-to-chair transfers as well as wheelchair propulsion. PTs also teach family members and other future caregivers transfer techniques and additional mobility tasks that will be useful at home. These therapists are also responsible for determining which specialty equipment, such as wheelchairs and leg braces, are most appropriate in a given situation.

The *occupational therapist (OT)* concentrates on the practical activities of daily living during rehab, such as grooming, bathing, eating, dressing, and toileting, as well as basic skills like upper-body strengthening and fine motor coordination that are necessary to carry out these tasks. OTs help with transfer training, especially to the tub and toilet, and also design and create splints for the upper extremities that help with positioning or in performing functional tasks like eating or writing. As patients become more functional, these therapists may also begin taking them into the rehab unit's makeshift kitchen to plan and cook meals or work on other household jobs like vacuuming and laundry.

Although not everyone with spinal cord injury needs the services of a *speech-language pathologist,* two groups of patients may: those with tetraplegia who have a tracheostomy or a halo brace; and those who have also sustained brain injuries at the same time as their SCI. Newly paralyzed individuals who need tracheostomies either have injuries to the highest part of the cervical spinal cord and are unable to breathe without a ventilator, or have cervical and high thoracic injuries that have paralyzed their chest muscles and weakened their ability to cough, making them prone to pneumonias.

Since patients are usually not able to talk with "trachs," speech therapists can help them develop alternate means of communication and practice swallowing exercises that might help them eventually regain the ability to eat. Many people who are in halo braces also have difficulty swallowing owing to their limited neck and chin movement; speech therapists help these patients find ways to make eating safer. Finally, those who experience brain injuries and have problems with memory or attention, for example, also benefit from speech-language services for cognitive retraining, which includes learning how to use memory strategies to compensate for their deficits.

Each patient is assigned a *case manager* (or *case coordinator*), usually a licensed social worker or a registered nurse by training. This individual handles all insurance and financial issues as well as discharge planning, including arranging home services or outpatient rehab therapies. Case managers often assist physicians by acting as the liaison between families and the interdisciplinary team, as well as helping arrange family meetings and training sessions.

Psychologists (or *neuropsychologists*) are available for supportive counseling for both patients and family members. When patients have difficulty following the rules of the rehab unit, for example, psychologists will often work with team members to design behavioral plans to improve the situation. For patients with traumatic brain injuries, neuropsychological testing may be necessary to determine the extent of damage and to help decide if individuals are ready to return to work or driving.

Therapeutic recreation specialists (or *recreational therapists*) help people with SCI develop new or adapted leisure activities, such as wheelchair basketball, fishing, or hands-free painting (in which people hold brushes in their mouths). Recreational therapists also collaborate with the other team members in arranging community outings to the movies, shopping malls, or sporting events.

When dealing with a challenging condition like spinal cord injury, the ability to discuss all aspects of a patient's care with professionals from different disciplines helps ensure that no detail is missed. This approach lets us take advantage of the knowledge and experience of the various team members, all of whom are focusing their efforts on the same long-term goal—teaching the patient how to resume life after his or her injury. Although each team member has an individual role, there is some overlap between services. Both nurses and therapists work on transfer training, for example, while *all* team members actively contribute to spinal cord education, support, and guidance for the patient and family. In every rehab facility, the interdisciplinary team holds weekly conferences to discuss the medical and nursing issues faced by patients, along with their progress in therapy. These meetings also give team members a chance to address concerns and work out possible solutions. In some cases, they may decide that therapists should visit a patient's residence and make recommendations regarding accessibility improvements to ease the eventual transition home.

Reactions and Reflections

"When I was first hurt, I was joking around and didn't realize the seriousness of it," says Bill, who sustained a C5-C6 fracture in a car accident as a teenager. "I didn't feel anything, so I thought I was fine. I don't think I even knew what a quadriplegic was. When I heard someone 'broke their neck,' I figured they died. That's the way it is in the movies and video games. It's nothing you can prepare for, no matter how much people think they can."

Like Bill, very few people have had any first-hand experience with disability or have known anybody who is paralyzed, beyond characters on TV or in the movies. So when an individual is first injured and arrives on the rehabilitation unit, he or she usually has no idea what it is like to be a person with spinal cord injury. Not being able to walk seems unimaginable; many assume that such a life could only mean complete dependence on others and never-ending obstacles and frustrations. People who are newly paralyzed frequently make false assumptions about their situations because they lack the knowledge that can come only through experience. Patients have often asked me and other team members how they will ever be able to work again or have a family. Some cannot imagine anyone ever accepting or loving them as they now are. A few have even asked if they will ever be happy again.

Although everyone goes through this process in their own unique way, initial feelings of loss and emotional upheaval are almost universal. First reactions are routinely negative; the shock of this unexpected event is often followed by an intense sense of tragedy or grief. Regardless of one's personality or background, a spinal cord injury causes almost everyone to question whether they have the strength to go on and, if they do, what will become of them. Understandably, family and friends will often try to talk an injured individual out of any despair, sadness, or grief. Yet these intense emotions, no matter how negative, are a natural part of the healing process. I have found that patients with the healthiest psychological adjustments are those able to work through their feelings and, just as important, have them validated by others.

The way loved ones react to an injury will also have a great impact on how the patient handles it. Families who possess a solid foundation of unconditional support and respect will usually try as hard as they can to assume as normal a life as possible. Instead of seeing SCI as a defeat, they will regard it as a battle to win. These are the people who educate themselves as much as they can about the possibilities; they search the Web, talk to other families on the unit, and look into community resources. One patient told me that his wife's steadfast involvement in his care pushed him to go to therapy even when he didn't feel like it. He didn't want to let her down; her persistence spurred on his own.

Some families and friends, in contrast, have difficulty handling the intensity of the situation. Too devastated to work with therapists to learn how they can assist in their loved one's care, they may even have trouble making regular hospital visits or watching therapy sessions. Whether they are fearful of the future when the patient returns home, or the incident has triggered fears and insecurities about their *own* health, their attitude can be detrimental to the individual with SCI. Well-meaning family and friends may inadvertently deepen a newly paralyzed person's sense of loss by responding with pity or sympathy. I have found that this kind of negativity stems from loved ones' misperceptions about life with disability. Still, it can be hard for the newly injured person to get past such pessimism.

No matter how concerned they may be, family members and friends should try to be positive and open-minded about what lies ahead for their loved ones—and themselves. Families are not expected to deal with SCI on their own; social workers, psychologists, and even hospital chaplains are available to help loved ones through this difficult period. Some people also find solace in talking to other families on the rehab unit about what they are going through, either on an informal basis on in a support group setting.

Experts have asserted that people with spinal cord injuries go through specific stages in response to their new disability, much like those experienced when a loved one dies. People are "supposed" to progress through an orderly sequence of reactions; it is also assumed that once they have passed all these stages, they will then be more or less adapted to their new life. Nothing, of course, is that simple. In my experience, people who are newly disabled have extremely varied responses. Each person goes through his or her own unique adjustment process, with or without a specific progression of stages. Some feel all the emotions at once; others go back and forth between phases; and still others seem to skip certain responses altogether. Because no two people face SCI with the same emotional, interpersonal, and cultural perspectives, there will always be more differences than similarities among the reactions.

Specific Reactions

Shock and Denial

Tommy, a rising high school basketball star, was involved in a motorcycle accident during his senior year. Lying on the ground while waiting for the ambulance, the seventeen-year-old could not feel or move his legs. The minutes felt like hours until the paramedics arrived—not because he was worried about a possible spinal cord injury but because all he could think about was being able to play in the sectional championship the next day.

Shock is a fairly common initial reaction to SCI, as the enormity of the situation prevents the injured or sick person from processing what has happened, both intellectually and emotionally. The individual seems to have no outward response to the news: he or she is simply numb. In such cases, people may need to rely on their significant others to help with gathering information and making decisions related to their care. Others will cope by breaking the specific issues down into manageable pieces and avoiding any focus on the "big picture" for the time being.

People who are unable at first to absorb the reality of their situation may respond next with denial. This defense mechanism is used to protect the mind when reality is too overwhelming to bear. Denial may be the only way that some people can continue to function and maintain their determination during rehabilitation and beyond. The loss of their physical abilities may just be too painful to handle early on.

Denial in certain forms can actually be a very effective means of coping with a difficult situation. It limits the amount of information a person has to process mentally, thereby making it easier for him or her to come to terms with the situation. It's almost like a means of buying time; denial serves as a way to preserve hope and keep a person's mind off the challenging aspects of life after SCI. At the same time, it can help patients maintain their optimism and motivation.

Roger, a forty-four-year-old man with C5 tetraplegia whose spinal cord was severely damaged in an industrial accident, continually insisted to his therapists that he would fully recover and "walk out of rehab." Despite this belief, however, he kept practicing transfers from his power wheelchair using a sliding board. It was his optimistic outlook and energy that enabled him to get out of bed and participate in physical therapy day after day. Roger didn't really envision his life with a wheelchair, but he was preparing for it just the same.

The degree and duration of denial varies, often depending on people's ability to cope. Some refuse to recognize the extent of their disability, while others will not acknowledge the permanence of their paralysis. Occasionally denial is so strong that people will not even remember what their doctors have told them about their injury or their prognosis: They fully repress any memory of the conversations. Others will be able to acknowledge that they have *had* a spinal cord injury but resist accepting the fact that their lives have forever changed as a result.

After the rupture of her aorta—the major artery that supplies blood to the legs and other organs—sixty-three-year-old Joann awoke in the intensive care unit paralyzed from her mid-chest down. After her transfer to a rehabilitation facility, she insisted that there was no

reason for her therapists to make a home visit to evaluate the acces-
sibility of her apartment. Only when she went home did she ac-
knowledge the reality: the front steps made it impossible for her even
to enter her building, and a ramp had to be built.

For some people denial is constant, while for others it waxes
and wanes. Most individuals do finally relinquish it, but usually
only when they are ready to move on in the grieving process and
begin adjusting to the changes. Others, however, remain in denial for their entire post-injury lives, never fully accepting the
permanence of their paralysis. This refusal to acknowledge reality often worries family and friends, but in most cases they
needn't be concerned—denial is what enables some people to
make it through each day. As long as they are still able to view
their lives as meaningful and worthwhile, denial "works."

On the other hand, denial may also prevent an individual
from acting in his or her own best interest. For example, a patient of mine with complete tetraplegia refused to be evaluated
for a wheelchair because he planned to walk out of rehab. Unlike Roger, who did learn to use a wheelchair even though he
maintained plans to walk, this patient did not have a positive response. I asked the team psychologist to work with him to develop a healthier perspective on the situation, and he eventually
agreed to the evaluation. Other patients have refused to attend
educational groups because they believe their injury is only temporary. Rather than attempt to change their opinion, I usually
encourage them to attend anyway as part of the program. "Who
knows," I say to them, "You might learn something that will be
helpful in one way or another."

Those in denial may also stay away from scheduled support
groups because they don't want to associate with disabled people, or avoid community outings that would mean being seen
using a wheelchair in public. Denial can not only prevent people

from fully benefiting from rehabilitation; at its most extreme it can also lead to self-neglect and secondary medical complications when individuals fail to follow recommended routines. This is the typical scenario for those who develop frequent pressure ulcers (commonly known as bedsores) from not turning in bed or shifting their weight when in a wheelchair. Denial can cause these people to be careless about their health maintenance, and can even keep them from obtaining proper medical attention when they are gravely ill.

If denial continues to be an obstacle, counseling from a mental health professional may be necessary to help these individuals expand their views of life with spinal cord injury—without causing the very despair they are trying so hard to avoid. When I have had a patient who is resistant to meeting with a therapist, I have often offered him or her the opportunity to meet with a peer visitor who has a similar level of paralysis and has already successfully made it through rehab and back to the community. In many cases, if the new patient is willing, the ability to hear real-life examples of how someone else got through rehab and "back to life" goes a long way to relieve uncertainty and fear. At the same time, this kind of one-to-one interaction may even result in these newly paralyzed individuals' participating more fully in the rehab process.

Some people fear that to give up denial and accept their situation would mean to surrender all hopes for recovery. In such cases I've tried to help patients understand that acceptance really means being able to recognize what is best for them *now*. Even when the expected outcome is not a full recovery, people with SCI never have to give up hope. Rather, they might redirect it; instead of dismissing anything short of walking out of rehab and back into their old life, they might hope instead that whatever the future brings, they can meet it with confidence and adequate knowledge. To this end, I encourage all newly paralyzed individuals to be as actively involved in their rehabilitation as possible; to learn about their injury and its effect on their bodies; and to participate in all their therapy sessions. Even when they believe that they will make a full recovery, I explain, it is always beneficial to understand as much as possible about their situation right now.

During rehab, it is normal for the person adjusting to a new spinal cord injury to waver between these two mindsets: one in which they expect to "walk out of here" and the other in which they plan to use a wheelchair for mobility. On the same day that Tommy talks enthusiastically about rejoining his basketball team for the coming season, for example, he may also attend an equipment clinic to be measured for the appropriate model wheelchair. Usually, as the newly injured become more knowledgeable about the possibilities of their future lives, their comfort level with their disabilities increases. Once this happens, they may be able to begin adjusting to the changes and developing a new understanding of themselves and their potential.

Anxiety

In the first few months post-injury, people often admit to high levels of stress. This seems to be especially true if the SCI was caused by a sudden, unpredictable, or violent event like a fall, bullet wound, or high-speed car accident. Suddenly, the injured person must worry about bowel and bladder accidents, accessibility, and even how to handle falling out of a wheelchair. Nightmares are common. Dependence on others, coupled with a perceived loss of control, further adds to an ever-increasing sense of uneasiness. Many newly paralyzed individuals voice concerns about being a burden to their loved ones; they worry about their loss of income and their ability to be effective spouses or parents. All at once, the future is uncertain.

These people need a chance to put their concerns aside and focus on learning ways to relax and manage their anxiety. The rehab psychologist is often the best person to teach such strategies, including meditation and proper breathing. Many patients find that by taking the initiative to work with the rehabilitation team and help plan their own treatment and goals, they are able to reestablish a sense of control over their situation. Learning as much as possible about one's injury can be another effective way to manage anxiety.

Anger

"I was pissed off for a while after my injury," says eighteen-year-old Jeremy, who became paralyzed after a diving accident. "Before, I was always kind of a laid-back guy who didn't let things bother me. But after I went to rehab, I'd get angry when I got UTIs [urinary tract infections] and got real sick. I'd start throwing elbows and stuff at the PTs. Some of the nurses would piss me off, too. If I couldn't do something, like learning how to cath myself, I'd throw the catheter on the ground. I knew I had to get over it, or I'd just be in bed all the time rotting, but I didn't know how."

Jeremy's response is especially common in those who are used to being strong, successful, and "in charge." Feeling powerless over their current circumstances, they may outwardly express rage to disguise these fears. When another person's actions or an unexplained disease are to blame for the paralysis, the anger is often even more intense.

This kind of fury is the emotional response to all the frustration they are feeling. The changes to be faced after injury may be overwhelming; for the first time in a person's life, he or she may have to ask others for help with the simplest of tasks. Irritation builds as the patient with SCI finds himself unable to scratch an itchy nose or get out of bed alone. It can be even worse when help involves the daily task of inserting a suppository or doing self-catheterization. For those who resent their situation and have difficulty acknowledging their need for assistance, anger often results.

Unfortunately, anger can be destructive and leave a person with an even greater sense of powerlessness and loss of control. During rehabilitation, hostility is often misdirected toward hospital staff. People have been known to yell at their therapists, refuse to get out of bed, throw equipment around the gym, and even engage in screaming fights with their loved ones. (Because family is always expected to "stick around," they are often on the receiving end of anger.)

Sometimes the target may just be any nondisabled person who reminds them of what they have lost. Whatever the case, the newly paralyzed individual will quickly come to learn that this kind of behavior does little to lessen the challenges of disability—and it usually alienates the very people he needs on his side.

"Every time I was in a bad mood in rehab, I'd yell at my mom," recalls Jeremy. "She would just say, 'I'm leaving!' and do it. I think that was good for me. I'd feel awful about it, and the next day I'd tell her I was sorry."

On the other hand, people who are unable to express or resolve their anger can become stuck in a cycle of loss, frustration, and depression, and may never learn effective ways to adjust to their disability. Ironically, those individuals who can express this same anger in a socially appropriate way often end up being the ones who experience the most psychological growth and positive change. Their frustration needs to be appropriately channeled, however, in order to positively redirect emotional energy and move forward. It was just this type of passion, born of anger and frustration, that gave countless paralyzed individuals and their loved ones the determination necessary to mount grassroots efforts that resulted in legislation such as the Americans with Disabilities Act (ADA) of 1990, which protects people from discrimination on the basis of their disability.

Sadness, Grief, and Depression

Although each person reacts to a spinal cord injury in his or her own way, almost everyone experiences feelings of sadness and grief. With all the loss and change, these kinds of emotions are only natural. Some feel tremendous guilt; others, deep regret. People may find that they are much more emotional than before their injury, with the slightest frustration now capable of triggering tears. Interest in food, sleep, and any pleasurable activity may dwindle.

Yet those individuals who can still talk about their sadness and grieve their losses openly will usually come to manage their discouragement and prevent it from interfering with their rehab and adjustment. In my experience with newly injured patients, I have found that most people respond best when their negative emotions are validated. They need to be reassured that the sadness and despair they are experiencing is "real" and "OK." Numerous losses *have* occurred, and they're not just physical: Patients also face diminished independence, control, societal status, job options, financial security, privacy, and many other aspects of life previously taken for granted.

Accordingly, people with new spinal cord injuries should be encouraged to express their unhappiness, even as they try to focus on what remains for them. They should be allowed to contemplate those things they can no longer do—like stroll on a beach or ride a bike. By doing so, they are able to keep alive memories of their previous experiences as a part of who they are and, at the same time, prevent the sadness from impeding their emotional recovery. This is a healthy part of the grieving process. In contrast, those who repress these types of emotions and don't allow themselves to experience them may have more difficulty moving on. When people avoid facing their losses, additional negative consequences like self-deception, substance abuse, and serious clinical depression can result.

When the grieving process *does* work, individuals are able to gain a realistic view of their losses and the impact that paralysis will have on their lives. At this point they are better able to find creative solutions to meet the challenges that their new disability presents. Once they are able to recognize their own innate abilities and potential, they are ready to regain control over their lives as well as manage any feelings of sadness or grief that may come along.

Despite the initial sadness and grief that accompany SCI, the good news is that, overall, most people with new spinal cord injuries will still be able to function and complete the tasks necessary to live day-to-day. During rehabilitation, for instance, they will continue to attend occupational therapy sessions to work on self-care skills like dressing; keep learning how to transfer from a wheelchair in physical therapy; and still visit with friends and family after therapy. They will usually respond positively to the support of others, and with extra encouragement, many will even agree to participate in community outings during rehab— even if it's without a smile. Individuals with this degree of sadness are still able to take responsibility for their lives, even if they may not feel up to the task at the moment. This ability to be redirected from their negativity, for however short a period, is what makes this group different from those who are more severely and *clinically* depressed.

For some people, feelings of worthlessness, self-blame, and

even death become pervasive. At this point, what was initially normal grief can escalate into clinical depression. Individuals in this situation are unable to function; their sadness becomes despair, and their feelings of inadequacy become self-pity. They are incapable of seeing *any* meaning in their lives or any ways to improve their situation. They may isolate themselves and ignore their health, subsequently developing medical complications like pressure sores or infections. Anyone who feels this way should be referred to a mental health professional for treatment of clinical depression. Help *is* available. With medications, counseling, or both, people can regain self-esteem and motivation and begin to move on with their lives.

At one time it was thought that some degree of clinical depression was a "universal" and even necessary part of the spinal cord injury experience. We used to think that intense sadness was a positive indication that a person recognized the implications of his or her injury. As such, depression was thought to signify the beginning of "adjustment." With this line of reasoning, individuals who did *not* become depressed after such a life-altering event were thought to be in extreme denial, unable to face their new reality. We now know, on the basis of many medical studies, that depression is not necessary for a healthy adjustment to spinal cord injury, and that many people return to productive, meaningful, and happy lives without ever feeling such intense sorrow or grief.

Day by Day: Tips for Helping Loved Ones Make It through Rehab

Few people go through rehabilitation entirely alone. It has been my experience that family members and friends are critical to the recovery process; in most cases their presence—or absence—has a tremendous impact on a newly injured person's ability to get through these first tough months. Patricia, the wife of one of my patients, remained by the side of her husband, Bill, each step of the way as he participated in rehab for a cervical spinal cord injury that he sustained in a fall while on vacation. Throughout the long weeks of his hospitalization, she was able to cope with the challenges and at the same time create many practical solutions to ease Bill's adjustment. As a teacher and writer, Patricia also had the foresight to record her experiences. In sharing them here, she hopes to help other families facing the same circumstances.

"In the blink of an eye," says Patricia, "a devastating accident happens to someone you care about, and because of it, change is thrust upon you. The transitions may be slight or immense, but how you all cope with them will determine whether they become positive challenges you can work through together or negative ones that weigh you down. At a time when so much seems out of control, you can control how you deal with spinal cord injury together.

"Just as each person perceives any situation in his or her own way, the effects of paralysis will have different implications for each family encountering them. You may endure arduous, demanding tasks and irretrievable losses, but you have a choice whether you live your today and all your tomorrows with dignity or with pity. You can't change what has happened. You can, however, choose to face your new challenges with courage, inner strength, and grace. Furthermore, you can decide to live each day with a sense of humor as an ally.

"Whether your loved one remains in the hospital for two weeks, two months, or longer, the experiences and emotions are similar. As the wife of one of my husband Bill's roommates said to me, 'It's like I'm standing still and the world is going on all around me.' You may feel like a spinning top because of the astronomical stress and fatigue, loneliness, hopelessness, anguish, and confusion. You are hag-

gard and weary and at times can hardly catch your breath. These feelings tend to diminish with time, but the fluctuating levels of stress do continue. Unwanted change and uncertainty are everywhere.

"During these moments of anxiety, it's important to remember two things: Because so much around you and inside you has changed, you are now stronger, wiser, and more blessed. You are also not alone. Friends and strangers alike care about what you and your loved one are going through. With empathy they will relate stories of aunts who broke legs or hips, underwent rehabilitation, and did well. You listen and nod, but you know it's not the same. Unless those people have experienced spinal cord injury with a loved one, they don't know what this life is like. It's an unmatched scenario.

"The following tips grew out of ideas that I worked out during my husband's lengthy hospital stay. Should you choose to use them, I hope they will lessen your apprehension and confusion, as well as lend some stability to your life while your own loved one is undergoing rehabilitation—and beyond."

At the Hospital

1. In the days after your family member's injury, record a message on your home voicemail with pre- and post-surgery updates. If you use e-mail, write an instant message with the same information that will automatically bounce back to people when they send you notes. Those who hear or read the latest message can pass it on. (In addition, internet-based programs like Carepages.com allow you to set up free, private websites where family and friends can go to read about a patient's progress and post notes and photos.)

2. Tape a list of important numbers by your phone—including your family member's hospital room, the doctor's

office and pager, and other relatives or friends you'll need to call quickly. If your cell phone stores numbers, make these your first numbered entries.

3. Designate specific people as central information agents, with duties to inform others about what's happening. Select one person from your loved one's workplace, one of his or her relatives, and one of your neighbors. Making five calls a day is far less taxing on you than constantly repeating an update to dozens of caring friends and family members.

4. When your friends ask if they can help, take them up on the offer. Be sure to delegate. One can vacuum your house, another can watch your children, and still another can do your grocery shopping or make you a meal. Somebody could even mow your lawn. Let each helper know what others are doing and encourage them to rotate duties.

5. If you don't work outside the home, plan to spend four days each week with your partner. You'll need the other days to do laundry, run errands, spend time with your children and/or close friends, make calls, exercise, or just rest. You also may be working with a contractor to make your home more accessible for your loved one—this, too, takes time.

6. Attend all educational meetings, support groups, team conferences, and other such sessions that the hospital arranges. These are for your benefit as much as for your loved one's well-being.

7. Keep a calendar on which to note your family member's daily ups and downs—medical, therapeutic, and emotional. He or she may not remember much of what goes on during this challenging period, but these records will enable you both to see what you went through. You'll also

have a log of events should a doctor need additional information, or should you need to address negative patterns. If you learn, for instance, that your family member always has a rough day after a particular activity or visitor, you can prepare for it.

8. Bring in an instant or digital camera and take pictures of your family member's slightest signs of recovery. Your loved one may need these photos as a way to see improvement, even if he or she cannot feel it. In addition, take fun, candid shots of the hospital staff and tape these around the room. They will give him or her a sense of boundary and the room a cheery atmosphere. Bring in old, fun pictures as well, and artwork by children, grandchildren, or nieces and nephews. This will help the room become a place people will want to visit—not avoid.

9. You might also bring in a roll of transparent tape for hanging pictures and cards; Post-It notes and a pen for writing yourself (and your loved one) reminders; a black permanent marker for labeling personal items; and a binder or accordion folder to keep all relevant materials that the staff gives you. Information from the hospital and other sources should be organized so it's together when you need it.

10. As soon as possible, give your family member a shoebox filled with "big boy's (or girl's) toys" such as a CD player with headphones; music and books on tape; and recorded messages or sounds from the children, grandchildren, pets, or birds in the backyard. Include a deck of playing cards, and ask the recreational therapist about getting a special cardholder.

11. Purchase shorts and pants made of Microfiber elastic waists and zippers that are two to three sizes larger than those your loved one typically wears, along with some big-

ger V-neck or button-down shirts. This material resists moisture and dries quickly; plus, the nurses will appreciate the larger sizes when dressing him or her. The therapists will also be grateful that this kind of fabric allows for easier transfers in and out of bed.

12. If possible, take public transportation to and from the hospital. A train or subway can be quite relaxing in this chaotic and ever-changing time. Purchase monthly passes for a discount rate, and bring a novel or daily newspaper along for the ride.

13. Look into different telephone plans that may reduce your bill over the next several months, as you're apt to be making many more local and long-distance calls. You may also wish to check on the other phone options you don't already have, such as voicemail and call waiting. As you start dealing with social services and other agencies, and begin exploring home modifications such as elevators or lifts, you may find yourself on the phone much of the day and expecting dozens of return calls. Purchase a few calling cards as well, both for home and for the hospital.

14. If you own a dog, ask hospital staff about visits. (Cats are usually not allowed in hospitals because they tend to carry more diseases than dogs.) Your family member and dog need each other during this difficult transition period. You may also want to bring home your loved one's dirty laundry and let your dog or cat sniff it. It may sound silly, but this practice could bring comfort to your pet.

15. Show your family member that you are handling everything well by looking "in control" during your visits. After presenting yourself well in front of your loved one, you can let go with his or her roommate's partner down the hall. This person is your ally and knows what you're going through. As time goes by, you will become more em-

powered and in control of your life again, but for now you should accept that this calamity is temporarily draining you.

16. Involve your family member in as many decisions as possible. Bring in the bills and checkbook and go through them together if this was the "old" routine. Respect your family member's opinions and ask if he or she is comfortable with yours. Major decisions like home modifications will take time to finalize, so discuss them early and often.

17. Your family member may become angry—very angry— at times. Ask what is upsetting him or her, and then try to accommodate these needs. If you think it's necessary, speak with a nurse or social worker. Try never to react to an outburst with one of your own. Such displays of temper will do neither of you any good.

18. Speak with your partner's case manager about social service agencies in your area, such as support groups and private-pay nursing companies. Call them for current information and request to be added to their mailing lists. Ask for other leads from these sources, being sure to obtain names. Some agencies provide immediate assistance, while others have waiting lists.

19. If your family member's spinal cord injury necessitates changes to your home or car, make no quick decisions. Think about the situation as a whole, then break it down piece by piece—weighing each part carefully. If home modifications are necessary, contact as many contractors as possible for estimates.

Adjusting to a condition like paralysis is not simply a matter of going through a precise sequence of stages. While a spinal cord injury frequently happens in only a second, it may take months or even years to adapt. It often takes many high and low points before people are able to come to terms with the loss and changes in their lives. When they do attain a more positive focus, the intensely negative feelings usually start to fade. Eventually, most injured individuals come to realize that they themselves have *not* changed, even though their physical abilities are now different. And though all my patients have experienced some sense of loss for years after their injuries, the majority of them adjust well to the changes that paralysis has brought to their lives. In fact, most tell me that they can't imagine their lives in any other way.

Consider, for example, one thirty-two-year-old patient who has C4 tetraplegia and no movement in his arms or legs. When I asked about his life several years after his diving accident, he replied: "Things could have been worse. I could have had a brain injury and be unable to talk with or recognize my family, or I could be dead." And even though he needs complete assistance for even the simplest of tasks, he added, "There are still people a lot worse off than me."

Over time, I have watched many people adopt similarly positive attitudes. Asked the worst part about being in a wheelchair, another young man with paraplegia told me, quite matter-of-factly, "I don't know—I've been in a chair longer than I was walking. For me, it's normal to use hand controls while driving. I can't imagine trying to drive with my feet. I can't imagine what it would be like to stand up. I think I'd be scared because my head would be too far off the ground. I'm very comfortable with a lot of things the way they are now. What's normal for an able-bodied person wouldn't be normal for me."

3

Adjusting to SCI:
The Return Home

After a car accident left her with T12 paraplegia, Tammy celebrated her eighteenth birthday in the rehabilitation hospital. Strong family support helped keep her spirits up during rehab, but when she returned home her mood changed.

"On a typical morning, my dad would come in, wake me up, and make sure I remembered to take my pills," she explained of those early days. "My sister helped me take my shower, and my mom took care of my bowels. The accident brought my younger sister and me closer together, but it was hard to deal with the fact that now I always had to have somebody with me. I got angry that she was only seventeen but could go out and do whatever she wanted, when she wanted, by herself, and I had to sit and wait until Mom or someone else came home and helped me up the ramp out of our apartment. We lived on a hill, so I couldn't take walks by myself anyway. My mom would try to cheer me up when she came home, but sometimes I felt really bad about being a burden on everybody."

Once someone returns home and is no longer within the "safe walls" of the rehab unit, the real adjustment to spinal cord injury begins. In the hospital, everything revolves around the disabled person and his or her new injury. Most needs are attended to; each problem solved; any questions answered. Paralyzed people in this setting are all treated the same—they are part of a group. As rehabilitation specialists, team members are so accustomed to the world of disability that little makes our heads turn. Yet when a person returns home, the reality changes: He or she must now find a way to reintegrate with family, friends, and the community at large.

Almost every inpatient I've known or cared for begins to experience increasing amounts of anxiety a few days before discharge from rehab. While the return home is usually eagerly anticipated through most of their hospitalization, as the date nears they begin almost to dread it: Discharge means facing all the unknowns awaiting them in the "real world." The physical return home is one thing; the psychological adjustment to life as someone with a spinal cord injury is another. Before this point, therapists usually visit the person's home and make various recommendations on how to improve the accessibility of the residence. Partners or loved ones complete training in how to help the newly paralyzed individual get in and out of the car, bed, or shower. Despite this preparation, patients who are about to go home suddenly start to ask lots of new questions. They frequently became quite anxious and often seem to lose much of the confidence they have worked so hard to gain during their long weeks or months in rehab. Just as so many people do at the onset of hospitalization, they often begin to wonder again if they can make it in the real world.

This sudden increase in anxiety has become even more prevalent since the 1990s, when medical insurance companies began to limit the number of days a patient could stay in rehab. This means less time, not only for learning how to use a wheelchair, but also for adjusting emotionally to SCI. Shorter hospitalizations and quicker returns to outpatient therapies and the community mean less time to incorporate a new disability into one's identity and to grow comfortable with it.

Further compounding the problem is the fact that insurance companies no longer allow patients to take overnight trips home before discharge to practice what they've learned in rehab. During my medical training in the early 1990s, patients used these opportunities to try out some of their newly learned techniques for eating, transferring in and out of their wheelchairs, and going to bed in their own home setting, as well as socializing with their families and friends away from the hospital. By taking this first "step," they were able to start getting a feel for whether they were indeed ready for discharge.

These overnights also allowed the patient's loved ones an opportunity to see if *they*, too, were prepared—both to live with and to start assisting in the care of the newly injured. The insurance industry seems to believe that if patients are able to leave the close monitoring and care of the medical staff for twenty-four hours, then they probably do not need further hospitalization. Furthermore, some insurance carriers no longer allow SCI patients to leave the rehab facilities with their families for even a few hours during the day. As a result, community outings with members of the therapy staff have now become the only way for many of the newly injured to leave the hospital grounds.

Although most people with SCI experience a period of excitement when they first return home, this is often followed by a repeat of the same emotions previously faced in the early days of rehab: sadness, resentment, anger, frustration, and anxiety. Even with all the preparation and therapies they have been through, the reality of no longer being able to do what they once could in this familiar setting can be hard to handle. More specifically, when in the hospital, using a sliding board to get from the bed to a wheelchair or to the toilet, or grabbing a "reacher" (a piece of adaptive equipment) to get a box of cereal from the cupboard shelf, may not be a big deal since your roommate and everyone else is also using them. But now, needing to have this special equipment in one's home may be a frustrating everyday reminder about what has been lost. The stairs one used to run up two at a time have become a steep, unattainable barrier, and the ramps that lie over them are yet another sign that things have changed. When a person watches his or her family or friends seemingly breeze through their day-to-day routines without need for adaptations, frustrations may only intensify.

"I didn't want to come home; I was used to nurses being around me 24/7, and I was worried, 'What if I get sick? What if something happens to me?'" admits Robert of his early days as a seventeen-year-old with tetraplegia. "I've adapted, but I'm still always telling my brothers how they take stuff for granted. It used to take me about two seconds to get dressed. Now I can't do it myself, and even with someone helping me it takes twenty minutes. It takes me forty-five minutes to shower. My whole day has to be mapped out."

Adjusting to the return home after SCI means not only dealing with the spinal cord injury itself but also confronting the way you view the world and your place in it. No one, of course, can maintain a positive attitude all the time, but learning how to adapt to one's "new normal" and push aside feelings of self-pity that may creep in is an important factor in post-injury adjustment. Sometimes just being able to experience the intensity of negative emotions is enough to allow someone to move forward and find solutions. The support of family and friends can be invaluable, but in the end the strategies individuals create for themselves will determine how well they are able to integrate back into society, as well as handle the challenges—and the looks—that are likely to come their way in school, the workplace, or wherever else they venture.

Different People, Different Adjustments

A person's long-term adjustment to spinal cord injury, like his or her initial reaction to it, is an individualized process. Whereas some people may readily adapt to life with disability, others have more difficulty coping. Although the physical changes resulting from paralysis should never be minimized, in my experience some people are actually *less* devastated than others when they lose their ability to walk. People who find personal fulfillment through matters of the mind and intellect—such as literature and art—may find it easier to cope with a life of physical limitations. Individuals whose personal identity stems from their athleticism or physical abilities, in contrast, may find the losses of paralysis much more difficult to manage. At the same time, I've found that physically oriented people are often the ones who challenge themselves to master adapted recreational activities like wheelchair sports—consider the rugby players of the 2005 documentary film *Murderball*—and this, too, helps make their transition to life in a wheelchair more acceptable.

People with SCI continue to demonstrate, time and again, that the extent of their paralysis is not a major determinant of how well they will be able to adjust to life with disability. For example, many people with tetraplegia, some of whom have no movement at all in their arms or legs, have been able to resume work or school (with the appropriate assistance), continue meaningful relationships while developing new ones, and maintain a high quality of life, just like people with paraplegia who have full use of their arms.

So many of my patients have shown that what matters most for a successful adjustment to spinal cord injury is what they *bring* to their injury more than the paralysis itself. In other words, a person's character, life history, intellectual and emotional resources, and degree of family and social support make the biggest impact on his or her ability to live a meaningful and happy life with paralysis. The next three stories more clearly demonstrate this theory.

Linda: A Positive Adjustment to Injury

Linda, a twenty-three-year-old law student, broke her back after she lost control of her car on an icy highway. Until that point in her life, she had always been a leader. She was very involved in her school and community, and, since her mother's unexpected death when Linda was fourteen, she had taken over much of the daily care of her two younger sisters as well. So while she was initially distressed when told at the hospital the extent of her injury, those same attributes that she had always displayed soon came to the forefront. She learned more about spinal cord injury and realized that she could still finish school with paraplegia, still proceed with her wedding planned for that summer, and even enjoy her honeymoon in Hawaii. So what if she had to use a wheelchair? With all these plans in her head, Linda was able to motivate herself in rehabilitation and work toward discharge back home to her fiancé—who remained committed to their life together.

Linda's history of effectively coping with stress, as well as her past success in relationships and school, has given her the skill set and confidence to handle this new personal crisis. At the same time, her ability to maintain a realistic view of the world, and of herself, has helped others around her to cope with the situation as well. She realized that some things in life cannot be controlled, and she drew on her personal strengths to handle what she could. People like Linda are usually able to gain the most from rehabilitation, successfully reintegrate into their communities, and maintain productive lives despite their disability.

Sylvia: A False Sense of Security

A widow for many years, seventy-two-year-old Sylvia enjoyed her simple life of playing cards with friends and visiting her grandchildren. For her, each day was predictable: she woke at the same time, ate the same breakfast, and took part in the same activities. This routine was important for her, as she disliked the unknown. To Sylvia, things were black or white, good or bad, but never both.

Unfortunately, this well-controlled existence was dramatically changed the day she went to the hospital for chest pain that she had been experiencing for several weeks. She was taken for a cardiac catheterization, after which she found that she was unable to get off the table or move her legs. She was rushed to the radiology department for a spinal MRI, which revealed a collection of blood around her thoracic spinal cord. The blood thinner that she had been given during the cardiac procedure had caused bleeding into her spinal cord tissue, and she was now paralyzed from the waist down.

Sylvia reacted to her spinal cord injury with intense self-reproach and depression. She wondered what she could have done to deserve this, and she spent her initial days of rehab lying in bed, refusing therapies. When she finally agreed to work with the neuropsychologist on the unit, he was able to help her gain a new perspective on her paralysis. Eventually her participation improved, as did her progress.

After two months of rehabilitation and a great deal of family education by the therapy staff, Sylvia was discharged to her home under the care of a visiting nurse and home therapists. Her daughter-in-law continued to check in on her daily and help with the shopping and cleaning, but she could rarely convince Sylvia to take a trip away from the house.

Individuals like Sylvia often have a tough time adapting to SCI. They tend to believe that good things happen to those who act justly, whereas those who do not are punished. This kind of attitude may be helpful for some people when coping with a world full of ambiguity, but it doesn't usually work well in situations like Sylvia's. Because she can't accept that there are things in life over which she has no control, she blames herself for her paralysis. As a result, she feels intense guilt, which can prove more disabling than the paralysis itself. Fortunately, with enough encouragement, people like Sylvia often come to accept the help and advice of others and benefit greatly from the assistance of mental health professionals. With this kind of support, and by learning various strategies to help them manage the uncertainties of life, they are frequently able to adjust their views and begin adapting to their new lives.

Mark: A Failure to Acknowledge One's Needs

By age twenty-seven, Mark couldn't imagine that any more bad things could happen to him. He was the middle son of a single mother, with a father who had abandoned the family when he was only two years old. During his childhood, Mark was frequently left with little supervision, and on other occasions he was physically abused by his mother's boyfriend. Later, as a teenager, he often skipped school and got into trouble with the police for petty theft or drug possession. Now a young adult, Mark was on his own: no girlfriend, no job, and no responsibilities. The night he and his buddies went out racing on their motorcycles, high on heroin, they were just looking for a good time. What Mark found instead was disaster. Failing to negotiate a turn correctly, he crashed his bike into a tree, breaking his back and becoming paralyzed.

The thought of never walking again was unimaginable for Mark. He refused to believe what his doctors told him and insisted instead that he would soon be able to return to his carefree, able-bodied life. In time he became extremely depressed and angry, and he would often yell at his therapists or hurl equipment around the gym. Because he believed that information about spinal cord injury and its potential complications did not pertain to him, he never attended the weekly SCI classes during rehabilitation.

After only five weeks, Mark decided on his own that it was time to leave the rehab hospital. Although his team felt that he could have benefited from additional rehabilitative training and education, he stood his ground and was discharged to home. Unfortunately, Mark's "freedom" was short lived; six weeks later, he was readmitted

to the hospital with infected pressure sores and a urinary tract
infection.

For individuals like Mark, whose lives have been filled with repeated disappointments and loss, rehabilitation can be quite challenging. Because he had seldom had others to rely on, Mark had grown accustomed to taking charge of things on his own. In the hospital, however, he was expected to put all his trust in a group of strangers, his multidisciplinary team, and depend on them and others to help him relearn such tasks as dressing and bathing from a wheelchair. Those who, like Mark, have a low tolerance for frustration and refuse to accept the issues involved with spinal cord injury often experience depression and anger during this period. Although drugs and alcohol may have been Mark's "answer" in the past, they are no longer an option in rehab.

Thankfully, rehabilitation facilities offer plenty of resources to address longstanding personal issues such as substance abuse and marginal social support, which can stand in the way of progress. Yet without the ability to respect authority or recognize what's in their best interest, people like Mark will frequently ignore such opportunities for help. These are usually the same individuals who go on to develop medical complications and maintain a low quality of life. They are also at risk for premature death, either from continued self-destructive behavior and negligence or, sometimes, from suicide.

When Coping Fails

Substance Abuse

Unfortunately, instead of seeking or accepting the appropriate professional help after their injury, some people—like Mark—

instead turn to drugs and alcohol as a way to lessen their emotional or physical pain and help them get through the day. This is especially common among those who used such substances as a coping mechanism before SCI, as well as those whose paralysis may have somehow resulted from such habits. I've also found that individuals who do not or cannot return post-injury to the jobs that gave them much of their daily structure, self-esteem, or means of supporting themselves or their families are more likely to turn to substance abuse.

Drugs and alcohol enable people to forget the stress and frustrations of living with disability, yet they also prevent them from taking the healthy step of feeling their grief. These substances can even become a substitute for socializing with friends and family, thereby intensifying the loneliness experienced by some newly injured individuals. But such attempts to escape depression and feelings of powerlessness usually only work for a limited time. The good feelings quickly wear off, leaving people to deal with reality. Those who continue to escape it, of course, risk becoming long-term addicts.

As with the able-bodied population, people with spinal cord injuries who abuse alcohol and drugs also frequently ignore their health. Paying little attention to diet and exercise, they tend to gain weight and lose muscle strength, both of which interfere with mobility and function. Sitting in a stupor for periods of time can cause joints to tighten and contribute to pressure sores, especially if the person fails to shift her weight frequently or stretch regularly. Because alcohol and drugs affect balance and coordination, people who abuse them are at higher risk for falls and physical injury. Inhaled substances like marijuana and tobacco can contribute to breathing difficulties as well as increased infections. (This can be especially problematic for an individual with tetraplegia who already has decreased respiratory function.) Moreover, these substances can interact with the medications normally prescribed for a person with SCI and result in potentially serious medical complications.

When depression is the primary reason for substance abuse, the best strategy is to focus on this underlying mood disorder. Appropriate counseling and/or medications can help people gain the personal strength and energy necessary to handle the challenges of disability in a more constructive way. As a first step, mental health professionals usually help patients to accept responsibility for their behavior and stop blaming everyone and everything else for their unhappiness. Next, they will encourage them to acknowledge their specific feelings, even the negative ones. The goal is to help people realize that only *they* can make their lives worth living, and that drugs and alcohol are not the way to deal with their pain.

Other factors besides depression can also put someone at risk for substance abuse post-injury. A history of abuse beforehand is the best predictor of who may turn to drugs and alcohol *after* paralysis. Someone who has used these substances as a way to avoid problems in the past is very likely to continue this "strategy" until some sort of intervention occurs. Moreover, the group with the highest incidence of traumatic spinal cord injury—that is, young men between the ages of eighteen and thirty-five—is also the group most likely to abuse drugs and alcohol. This cohort also tends to be impulsive and drawn to thrill-seeking behavior, two more qualities that increase a person's risk for both spinal cord injury and substance abuse.

In general, treatment for substance abuse among people with SCI should focus on ways to foster independence, build self-esteem, and help the patient return to a productive and healthy lifestyle. Some individuals will need training in disability coping; others will need to relearn basic living skills. For those whose drug and alcohol problems predate their spinal cord injury and are more a result of ingrained patterns of behavior or family history than depression, a more traditional addiction treatment approach like Alcoholics Anonymous may be most appropriate. In such cases, the key is to recognize the risk factors and warning signs before they get out of control. A primary care physician may be a helpful resource for locating mental health professionals who have particular expertise with addiction. Although there are no known organizations specifically devoted to substance abuse issues in the disabled community, mental health counselors and others can provide information about available programs to treat addiction as well as accessible halfway houses for those in recovery post-injury.

Suicide

Further underscoring the importance of recognizing and properly treating clinical depression in individuals with SCI is the fact that suicide is becoming a major cause of death among this group. Studies cite the suicide rate for this population at anywhere from two to six times that of the general public, especially during the first three years post-injury. Although we might assume that degree of disability would predict tendencies for suicide, research does not support this. In fact, one study demonstrated that people with paraplegia experienced deeper depression immediately after rehabilitation than those with tetraplegia. It is important to note that many people with ventilator-dependent tetraplegia are happy to be alive and enjoy a high quality of life.

The risk factors for suicide after SCI remain the same as for those who are not disabled: previous episodes of depression; a history of substance abuse and a return to this habit post-injury; prior suicide attempts or a family history of such behavior; and limited social support. Whether paralyzed or not, people with these risk factors may have a limited ability to handle major life stresses. If they feel they have no one to turn to, they may view their situation as hopeless and see death as their only option.

It is crucial to keep in mind that suicide is not always a sudden event. Although a gun or pills are frequently used to accomplish the task quickly, it can also be slow and insidious from self-neglect, substance abuse, and the malnutrition, infections, and other lethal medical complications that often result from these behaviors. The key to preventing this tragic event is recognizing the risk factors—particularly the presence of depression—as well as helping those most at risk to get appropriate treatment as soon as possible. Families should understand that they are not in this alone.

Identifying Risk Factors for Clinical Depression

Because not everyone will be able to cope effectively with their new disability at all times, it is especially important to identify who may be at risk for clinical depression after spinal cord injury. As noted, the best predictor of whether a person may become depressed after paralysis is how he or she previously coped with life's demands. More specifically, individuals who have struggled with depression in the past, especially in response to intense stresses or life changes, should be closely monitored post-injury for any significant alterations in appetite, sleep, energy level, and mood. The same is true for those with pre-injury histories of substance abuse.

A family history of depression will also raise a person's chances of developing this mood disorder after paralysis. Some medications, such as diazepam (Valium) or lioresal (Baclofen) for spasms and narcotic analgesics for pain, may cause mood changes and can either result in or complicate depression as a side effect. Additionally, many of these same drugs have the potential to be abused, which could perpetuate the vicious cycle of addiction and depression.

Environmental factors can also contribute to depression after a spinal cord injury. These include financial resources, living arrangements, work life, and leisure pursuits, as well as access to transportation. Some people become understandably over-whelmed by the need to rethink so many aspects of their lives in the aftermath of spinal cord injury. Will I be able to keep my job? Will I have to move out of my home? Who will care for my chil-dren? In reality, though many of these obstacles seem insur-mountable, they can be tackled with some support, knowledge, and persistence. Many organizations and resources are available to help individuals with SCI and their families address these very issues, as we discuss in later chapters.

The other good news is that even with some of these risk fac-tors, many people are still able to cope with the changes in their lives after SCI and *never* become clinically depressed. Studies have shown that the presence of a supportive network of family, friends, and community resources is associated with a reduction in post-injury depression. The involvement of loved ones can help reinforce a person's self-worth, as well as his or her motiva-tion and hopes for the future. Similarly, for some patients, sheer gratitude at having survived may be enough to keep their spirits even, especially when paralysis may have resulted from a serious accident. In other cases, a person's role in the family—say, as the parent of several children, or as a new bride—enables him or her to stay positive and motivated. Setting goals like returning to work or school (to be discussed in Chapter 4) is yet another way people cope with the many challenges of spinal cord injury.

Studies and real-life examples continue to show that the risk for depression after paralysis is markedly lower for those who are able to make productive use of their time, either by socializ-ing with others, participating in leisure activities, or returning to some form of paid or volunteer work. The personal satisfac-tion and self-esteem that result often help to counter any sadness. Similarly, I have found that individuals who believe in their ability to control their own lives and to make things happen for themselves are also less likely to become depressed. Effective problem-solving skills and self-confidence help dampen any negative emotional responses to disability.

After rehab for a C5 spinal cord injury, Cindy Purcell moved back in with her mother. "She wanted me in the house and was determined to do my care," she recalls. "That just didn't work. It's my mother, you know? I used to hear her on the phone breaking plans like going shopping and saying, 'I can't do that; I have Cindy.' I became an excuse for her, and I hated that. So I called the Visiting Nurse's Association, and they came out to see me. They couldn't do my bowel care, my catheter, and my meds—I still needed Mom for that—but they did help me with bathing and dressing. It was a first step.

"Later I left the house and moved in with my boyfriend, who became my caregiver. That was also a mistake; we broke up, and I moved back home again. But this time I made the downstairs of my mother's house into an apartment, and got involved with the PCA [personal care assistant] system through the local Independent Living Center. I discovered that you could hire PCAs to do anything, and you were the boss. That was a great source of independence to me—I was finally back in charge of my own life."

Effective Coping Strategies

No matter the level of paralysis, a spinal cord injury is always a shock to a person's sense of self. Disability forces an individual to look at his or her life and rethink values, beliefs, and goals. For many, this type of soul-searching is an entirely new concept. Accepting membership into the disabled community is not an easy process and can take a great deal of time. Patients have told me that the best way to adjust to all the major life changes that come with paralysis is by experiencing them day-to-day. Only then are they able to separate the myth surrounding disability from the reality.

By adopting a positive attitude and rejecting the unsubstantiated negativity surrounding SCI, some people are actually able to view their injury and their reaction to it as a means of *improving* their lives—not just as a total loss of their former selves. This traumatic event may even empower them to begin reevaluating their aspirations. Patients tell me that once they are able to grieve for their old lives, they find themselves focusing on what still remains and what is possible for them, rather than dwelling on what they have lost. Their self-esteem is no longer tied to whether they can walk or use their arms; now it is about who they are, what they can contribute to society, and the lives they can touch.

A person will know he is on the right path toward adapting when he can acknowledge that, despite all the changes, he is still the same human being he was before his injury. He comes to realize that having a spinal cord injury does not mean that he is "sick" or that he will always need medical care; it means only that he is disabled. At the other extreme are individuals who choose to use their injury as an excuse to give up all responsibility. They readily accept the sympathy and assistance of others and never try to increase their own abilities. As time passes, they find it increasingly difficult to break this cycle of dependence. As a result, they may *never* learn to fully cope with disability and live up to their true potential.

Still, people who have effectively adapted to disability recognize that though certain aspects of their lives have become more challenging, they are far from ruined. Being paralyzed does not prevent them from dating or forming relationships, getting a college degree, securing a job, expressing themselves artistically and athletically, or finding other means of fulfillment (see Chapters 4–6). While such accomplishments may now require a little more time, creativity, and assistance, these individuals have the motivation to put forth the effort. Being paralyzed becomes just one more part of who they are, not their entire existence. SCI is "something they possess," not their whole identity; they are, for example, "people with paraplegia" rather than "paraplegics."

"Because I was always so accepting of my injury, I've had psychologists tell me I was in denial," says Meredith *of the attitude that has helped her get back to work and have two children after a spinal cord injury. "What actually happened was that I realized very early on what being paralyzed was going to do to my life. I didn't like it very much, but the way I looked at it, I had no choice. This is what had happened, it had happened for a reason, and maybe the reason would become clear to me at some point in the future."*

Focus on the Positive

I find that in addition to accepting life as it's now constituted, people with SCI do best when they're able to maintain the right perspective about the adjustments that must be made as a result of their paralysis. For example, while some individuals with tetraplegia may initially feel self-conscious about eating with specialized equipment like a wrist splint or plate guard (which keeps food from falling off the dish), eventually many of them come to realize that these devices allow them to enjoy eating without having to be fed; in that respect, they're a means to independence (see Figure 3).

With time, most disabled people do come to appreciate the value of adaptive gear and how it can help them regain their skills and independence. The same is true for the use of a wheelchair or other mobility aides. Those who have come to terms with their paralysis are usually able to regard their wheelchair as

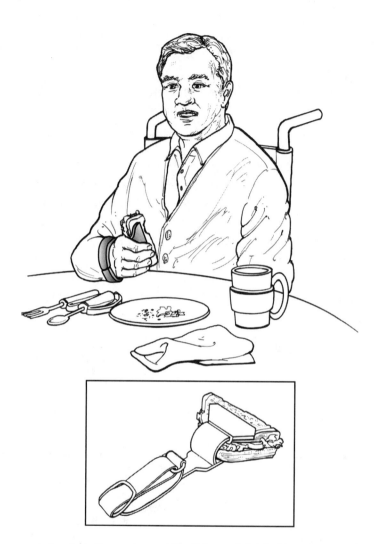

FIGURE 3. Adaptive equipment like this sandwich holder, spoon, and fork offer individuals with spinal cord injury increased independence in eating, dressing, and other activities of daily living.

a means to get from one place to another rather than as a symbol of their inability to walk.

Likewise, people with high tetraplegia or other injuries that require the assistance of a personal care attendant are often able to recognize that some *dependence* is necessary for them to gain a certain degree of *independence*. More specifically, they may realize that having a PCA to help with bathing and dressing each morning is a kind of "positive" dependence, that is, something that will, for example, enable a young woman with tetraplegia to get to her office each day and continue her job as a social worker. Accepting the need for some assistance often allows disabled people to maintain their overall independence.

"My motto is that 10 percent of life is what happens to you, and 90 percent is how you handle it," says Danny of the road he took to adaptation and acceptance after a car accident left him with paraplegia. "I had to work on bringing Danny back into my life after my injury. It took a lot of work with a psychiatrist to understand and develop the philosophy I've forged that my wheelchair is a piece of furniture. Spinal cord injury does not define me or control me. It has nothing to do with the person I am, day in and day out. My wheelchair helps me get from Point A to point B. That's it."

As I've seen many times with my own patients, hope is another crucial ingredient to coping successfully with spinal cord injury. Research has demonstrated that people who maintain adequate levels of hope experience less emotional distress, regardless of how much time has passed since their injury. This is a delicate balance, however; too much hope can bring intense disappointment if it's unrealistic, whereas the other extreme—despair—can be equally destructive. While some disabled people do center their entire lives on the wish for a complete cure, this is not the only kind of hope open to them. Some individuals aspire to making substantial progress during rehabilitation, to finding work, to falling in love, and to enjoying many more aspects of a fulfilling life than just regaining the ability to walk. When accepted and believed, this perspective on hope frequently provides a person with the strength to work through whatever grief, anger, sadness, and frustration he or she may be experiencing post-injury. And once these feelings can actually be managed, a person may very well be able to set new goals and remain determined to reach them.

There will always be some people who adamantly refuse to accept their paralysis. They feel that to do so would mean that they are *content* with their disability. But I believe there's another way of looking at "acceptance." This term can also refer to a person's refusal to let a wheelchair or weakened limbs interfere with his or her quality of life. At this point, which many of my patients have reached, an individual recognizes that while changes have to be made, life goes on. As a result, he or she can now take the first steps toward creating a different but no less meaningful and productive life after paralysis.

It is no surprise, then, that studies have shown that people who possess personal goals that keep them motivated adjust well after SCI. Such aspirations are different for everyone and usually depend on a person's life history and current circumstances. Furthermore, such goals will likely change several times through the years. For most people, aspirations and dreams give life purpose. For the newly injured, the challenge of getting through inpatient rehabilitation and returning to one's home often motivates them to persevere. In other cases, they are driven by the desire to enjoy a favorite leisure activity or find satisfying employment again. The dream of being a parent (see Chapters 8–9) can also be a powerful incentive to ride out the tough times and forge ahead. But no matter the goal, people who feel like they have something to live for are usually more likely to adapt to their disability and move forward with satisfaction and happiness.

4

Back to Productivity:
Work, School, and Play

Textbooks state that the goal of rehab is to help individuals "achieve the fullest possible psychological and physical adjustment to their disabilities," but the truth is that what we're really trying to do as physicians, nurses, and therapists during this period is get people back to *life*—the most productive life possible. For some, this will mean going back to work; for others, caring for their children; and for still others, returning to school or a favorite pastime. In many cases it will be a combination of things. The point is that once people have learned to manage the physical aspects of paralysis during rehab, it's time for them to start educating themselves and thinking about how they will fill their days after discharge.

I have certainly seen the benefits of continued productivity after SCI: Those patients who have returned to the workplace or resumed their educational goals are undoubtedly the happiest and most well adjusted. These are the individuals who have been able to redefine their lives despite disability and have not let their spinal cord injury define *them*. Returning to work or school has given them multiple benefits besides just a salary or a diploma. Rejoining the community means the chance for increased social contact, mental stimulation, and challenge, as well as a greater sense of purpose and achievement. It also lends structure to the day, something that many people miss after leaving the rehab unit with its regularly scheduled activities. In fact, the heightened satisfaction that they gain from "being useful" ends up positively contributing to other aspects of their lives, including family, health, and finances. In my experience, those who keep themselves busy and productive are also the least likely to turn to drugs and alcohol to fill in the gaps.

Undeniably, numerous challenges exist for people with spinal cord injury who decide to take these first "steps" back to life. Although the Americans with Disabilities Act (ADA) of 1990 made discrimination against such individuals in the workplace or elsewhere illegal, more subtle forms of inequity—and ignorance—still exist in interviewing and hiring practices. Moreover, once on the job, disabled people often have to contend with additional obstacles, both physical and emotional. Many buildings and transportation systems are now accessible, but some still are not; coworkers or fellow students often take the time to understand the needs of disabled colleagues, but some may be too uncomfortable or insensitive to even approach them. And while getting ready each morning and commuting to and from work can be a hassle for anyone, the time and effort involved are especially pronounced for those who need the help of a PCA and/or a wheelchair.

This chapter explores some of the various paths that people with SCI have taken back to work, school, and play, and how they've chosen to deal with obstacles along the way. You'll read stories about different individuals, including some of my own patients, who have charted new courses for themselves by learning additional skills on the job, returning to school, or tackling an entirely new trade or hobby. From the business student who realized after his injury that his true calling was teaching, to the firefighter who transferred her love for helping others into a new career as a peer counselor, these people have shown the resiliency and adaptability necessary to move forward after paralysis. We'll also hear from experts in the field of vocational rehabilitation, who will help shed some light on the potential logistical and financial challenges that these individuals face along the way. They will also offer tips on how to make the most of the growing opportunities and assistance available to those with disabilities.

Getting Connected: More Options Than Ever

When thinking about going back to work or school, most people with new spinal cord injuries have no idea where to begin. As vocational rehabilitation counselor Kathy Grady notes, "The thing that most worries hospitalized individuals and their families in the first weeks and months after an injury is how they'll handle the strain of rehab and recovery—especially the financial hardships. When you see patients and families in the hospital setting during this period, they're still being acclimated to their injuries and the changes in their lives. It's premature for them to think about their future in terms of returning to work. They don't know where their heads or bodies are yet—but they have lots of questions and concerns."

Rehab hospitals are mandated by CARF (the Commission on Accreditation of Rehabilitation Facilities) to employ a vocational rehabilitation counselor (or VRC) to educate patients and families on federal, state, and local resources that address finances, health insurance, employment, and educational concerns. Many of the questions frequently heard include: How am I going to afford help when I get home, since I'm no longer working? What health insurance is open to me now? Are there other means of financial assistance available from the state? My injury occurred on the job; am I entitled to workman's comp coverage? I'm paralyzed because of an accident, and there is a lawsuit—how much of any settlement will I have to give back to the state in taxes or litigation costs?

Now that insurance companies have changed reimbursement for rehabilitation hospitals, leading to shorter stays for patients, some newly paralyzed people are returning to the community after only six to eight weeks. As a result, the focus of the VRC has changed. Most counselors like Grady provide education and referrals to community resources. The first step is assessment of a patient's status, diagnosis, age, education, work history, and so on. Armed with this information, the counselor can then provide education about the government programs available to help those with disabilities.

Although services vary by state, two federal programs are available nationwide through the Social Security Administration (SSA): Social Security Disability Insurance (or SSDI) and Supplemental Security Income (or SSI). Claimants who have previously worked and meet SSA criteria for eligibility can apply for SSDI coverage, while those who are ineligible for the former, yet meet SSA's asset criteria, can receive SSI assistance.

For those who will need a personal care attendant (or PCA) to help with activities of daily living, vocational counselors will also explain how to contact the local Independent Living Center (ILC) to arrange for an assessment. These organizations grew out of the Independent Living Movement in California in the early 1970s and are run mainly by people who are themselves disabled, with the aim of helping those with SCI and other disabilities reconnect with the community. ILCs assess a client's functional abilities, then recommend to the state health insurance plan (for example, Mass Health for Massachusetts)—which provides the payments for personal care attendants—exactly how many hours of PCA assistance will be needed by the individual once he or she has returned to the community. Because standard health insurance companies will only cover home care for a specific time period, assistance from the state health insurance plan for PCAs (who in Massachusetts in 2007 earned nearly

$11.00 an hour) is imperative. The experts at Independent Living Centers also advise consumers on how to hire PCAs they can trust, as well as when it makes sense to find a new attendant.

Although various resources exist in the rehab setting to help with many aspects of life after discharge, patients must still take the initiative and learn as much as they can about what their community has to offer. As vocational rehabilitation counselor Grady explains, "We're always trying to get across to patients that they need to use community resources to help them rebuild their lives. Vocationally, the newly injured and their family go through a number of stages before they are truly capable of returning to community living."

This is the same approach I take with patients and families. But as much as we work to prepare them, it is only after they leave us and return to their new or old homes that reality sets in. They no longer have the structure of the hospital, with people looking out for and taking care of them each minute of the day. They need to find out what's available to them largely on their own. Doing so takes a lot of initiative, support—and courage.

Back to Work: Making the Most of Vocational Rehab Services

Accessing Services in the Community

Most newly paralyzed people are unable even to imagine the prospects of job hunting, let alone going on an interview. In the early days after injury, they are still learning how to manage a curb or just put on a suit jacket or pantyhose from a wheelchair. Once these skills are mastered, however, it's time to start thinking about how they will move forward.

When a person is emotionally and physically able to start thinking about a return to work but is either unable to go back to a previous job or needs help finding a new one, he should contact the Vocational Rehabilitation Services system for his state of residence. Sometimes rehab hospitals will directly connect individuals with a vocational rehab counselor, but if not, these professionals can easily be found through the Independent Living Centers and the state's Office of Health and Human Services. Once a meeting is arranged, the disabled person should be prepared to answer questions regarding his or her work history, education, any special job-related skills, and criminal record, as well as to provide details about his or her injury and any complications. (See your state's Vocational Rehabilitation website for more details on the information required.)

Once the VR counselor (VRC) has gathered all the data and asked the injured client about goals and employment expectations, he or she will then determine which state-funded vocational services a person may be eligible for on the basis of their capabilities. This process usually takes sixty days or less, after which the applicant will be notified of their eligibility and priority category, which is based on the severity of injury as well as the potential barriers to employment. (Those with spinal cord injury usually qualify for the highest priority level and the full range of VR services.) Although many state-funded insurance plans will cover a portion of this employment-related assistance, sometimes the job seeker or his or her family will need to pay part of the cost. (An appeal process exists for those who believe their eligibility assessment is inaccurate.)

Once eligibility has been decided, the actual work of finding a job can begin. The VRC and client will together complete a vocational assessment to establish a career goal based on interests, personal strengths, education, and work history. Several meetings may be needed to map out a complete strategic plan, as well as to conduct additional vocational testing. In most cases, once the counselor and the client agree on a job goal, the next step is to develop an Individual Plan of Employment (IPE) for the job seeker. This document comprises a person's employment goal, his or her responsibilities toward reaching it, and the ways in which VR services will assist. Once completed, it serves as the guide for the weeks and months to come as the two parties continue their meetings in order to design a resume, discuss job openings, and prepare for interviews.

Cindy Purcell of the Massachusetts Rehabilitation Commission (MRC) is a vocational rehab counselor who has a good sense of what her clients are going through. Of the roughly twenty counselors working in the MRC's Worcester, Mass., office, Purcell is the only one who is disabled herself. At the age of eighteen she was involved in a car accident that resulted in tetraplegia. Purcell returned to school and after seven years secured a job with her local Independent Living Center as a transitional housing coordinator. She then joined the advisory council for the MRC, eventually lobbying for and earning a staff position with this state-run organization.

Like many of the people she now counsels, Purcell admits to having felt apprehensive when she started her new job in 1987. "I was really nervous; at the center I had been one of several disabled people on staff, but at the MRC I was all alone," she recalls. "Since I didn't know anybody, I worried whether they would accept me for who I am. I had all kinds of concerns. Who was going to help me get my lunch and get my silverware out? If my leg bag got full, who could I ask for help? And what if I had a foot spasm and my feet fell off my wheelchair?

"Fortunately, I'm outgoing and could make friends easily," she continues. "It took me a few days to feel comfortable, and I made sure not to drink too much so my leg bag wouldn't fill up. It's not another person's job to help you with something like that unless they know you really well. You either have to arrange to have a PCA come in, or you need to work on networking with people as much as possible so you can make friends and feel okay asking for help."

Twenty years later, Purcell oversees a caseload of more than 140 clients and meets with roughly 7 of them daily. "Some of them have worked before, others haven't, but the end goal is always getting back to work and back to functioning in society. There are a lot of hurdles people come up against. They may have substance abuse problems, be in recovery from depression, or just have a lack of independence or motivation. When I'm talking with companies seeking workers, I focus on describing a client's abilities while at the same time trying to get a feel for if he or she can do that particular job. You need to make sure it's a good match, and of course you need to make sure the workplace is accessible to that person's needs."

Purcell's clients grapple with other challenges as well. "Many people seem to have difficulties with personal care attendants," she says. "Sometimes they have problems with them stealing from them or not showing up—and this, of course, impacts their own employment situation depending on how much they need a PCA to get ready and out the door to work each day. If they are able to drive, we can help them get access to vans. If they can't drive themselves, we can help find them a van service or a bus line that stops by their house and can take them near their job. As much as experience or skills, a person's commuting situation may impact which jobs he or she is able to handle."

The key to success during all stages of vocational rehab is open communication. If at any time a client feels that his or her needs are not being met through the services delivered, the counselor should be told about it. If a problem still can't be resolved, the client can always meet with the counselor's supervisor. In fact, the Client Assistance Program, mandated under the Rehabilitation Act of 1998, was specifically devised to help with such complaints. Bear in mind, however, that a time limit often exists for appealing any change or denial of vocational services.

In some cases, individuals may need to do more than just work with a VR counselor to find a job. For example, an injured person may lack the confidence needed to advocate fully for himself; he may not feel capable of speaking up when he feels a position isn't the right fit or if a counselor is not pushing for him strongly enough. In these cases, the job seeker's local Independent Living Centers may be able to provide the extra help necessary. ILCs are located in most major cities and many smaller ones, too. They serve as advocacy centers where people can receive peer counseling as well as help learning independent living skills.

For example, if a person is having difficulty connecting with her VR counselor, support groups at ILCs are available to provide reassurance and tips on ways to handle the situation. Many of the centers also have their own job banks and vocational counseling services. In neighborhoods plagued by violence, these organizations can additionally serve as safe havens for the growing number of young people paralyzed through acts of brutality and left to fend largely for themselves after rehab.

Making an Impression: The Interview

Once a person finds a position that interests him, the next important step is a successful job interview. The VR specialists help clients develop the proper interviewing skills through coaching, role-playing, and multi-media presentations. Making a strong impression is especially crucial for applicants with SCI, who can face subtle (and at times unintentional) prejudice from employers when they meet for the first time. Some job seekers with paralysis have told me that they believe the best way to get interviews is to focus attention *away* from their disability as much as possible. For example, when writing cover letters or calling to set up meetings, they won't even mention their injuries to prospective employers to prevent any possible bias.

Although this approach may seem a sensible way to ensure that you are evaluated strictly on professional merit, it can also be risky. Some employers—even the least judgmental—may be so genuinely taken aback by seeing a candidate show up in a wheelchair that the whole interview process is thrown off. Then there is the possibility (experienced by several of my patients) that a disabled candidate will arrive at a meeting only to discover that the site is not accessible. Chances are, if you can't get up the stairs or through a doorway to a potential workplace, you're certainly not going to be in the best frame of mind for an interview.

Given these scenarios, most vocational rehab counselors will recommend that a job candidate be clear and honest on the phone about his or her disability once an interview has been secured. In addition to eliminating any unwanted surprises (like an inaccessible venue), such candor will also minimize the chances for awkward moments at the in-person meeting. Likewise, a confident approach to the interview itself will also be beneficial. "You hear about employers clamming up and just staring at the applicant's wheelchair," says counselor Cindy Purcell. "We tell our clients to be up front and make sure to put the interviewer at ease. You need to be the person in charge to make the situation comfortable.

"For example, even if you have tetraplegia, be sure to extend your hand if you can—and don't worry if the interviewer is apprehensive about taking it," Purcell adds. "Just tell them flat out, 'I was in a car accident (or whatever the case may be). I use a wheelchair, but I can do the job.' If you don't say anything, you can bet the interviewer is still going to be wondering the whole interview why you're in the chair. It's human nature. So you might as well get it out in the open. In twenty years of helping people get ready for interviews, my experience has shown me that when people are candid, they usually get the job."

Of course, some of the most sensible strategies for obtaining a job interview—and the job itself—are the same no matter what a person's physical abilities. Resumes should be routinely updated and uncluttered. Informational interviews with individuals and companies of interest, even if they don't have openings, are a great way to get a feel for the process and leads on other opportunities. Once you schedule an interview with a prospective employer, practice a quick "personal sales pitch" in which you highlight the qualities that set you apart from other candidates. Dress neatly; your appearance is one way to show respect for an interviewer. Many colleges and high schools maintain excellent alumni banks; calling up an alumnus is a great way to break the ice and learn more about a particular job. If you have difficulty securing interviews, you might consider advertising your services in print or in online publications; joining job-networking groups can also be helpful. For surprisingly little money, these options can get word of your interest and skills out to a lot of people quickly.

Despite the best intentions and preparation, however, some individuals with SCI—like *all* potential job seekers—will still encounter frustration and prejudice on the job hunt. VR counselors like Purcell, as well as clinicians like myself, have heard numerous horror stories about interviews gone bad because employers are unable to look past wheelchairs at the people sitting in them, or ask completely ignorant or even offensive questions during meetings. Some of those tales are included in the pages that follow, but it's important to remember that, in the end, these people have all persevered; they have all not only gotten jobs but also thrived in them.

If a person is considering a return to her old line of work, the counselor, often with the assistance of a former employer, will sometimes create "job stations" to see if the job seeker still possesses the skills required to perform the necessary tasks. These simulated work environments can also help improve the worker's ability to perform the specific job with her new impairments and, subsequently, boost the client's confidence. If, during the job search, the client finds that potential employers are hesitant to hire someone with disabilities, the vocational counselor can step in and advocate for the client's abilities and potential.

Once a position is offered, job-site modifications may be needed. Here, too, the vocational rehabilitation specialist can be of assistance. Accommodations may include changes in the work schedule to allow a disabled employee extra time to get in each morning, as well as alterations in the physical environment to make it wheelchair-accessible. Modifications can be as simple as raising the height of a desk or as high-tech as adding computer software that will allow a person with tetraplegia to use voice recognition for data entry. Offices with stairs may need ramps, while those with community bathrooms may require designated areas where a worker can tend to his bladder program in private.

Yet even when an interview goes well and a candidate with SCI receives a position, on-the-job challenges may still arise as a result of his disability. For this reason, many people will choose to continue their relationships with VR counselors well after their "official" time together is over. This continued contact allows them to discuss any concerns that may arise and also increases the likelihood that the disabled worker will remain on the job for the long term.

"Some people need help with job stability," says Cindy Purcell. "Although their case is closed after ninety days, we remain here for them. One thing clients are always asking me is the same thing I was worried about—how to ask people for help on the job. I just tell them they need to form relationships. Attitude makes a big difference. One client took a job, and starting on the first day she demanded that somebody get her lunch, and of course nobody wanted to help her. You need to make your own way; that's the reality of life."

Purcell speaks from experience. She still remembers how fearful she was about asking able-bodied colleagues for help with her leg bag, but she also knows that her ability to be frank about her post-injury travails and achievements has been a big reason for her successful career as an advocate for others with disabilities. In fact, her first job after her accident was as a skills trainer at an independent living center, helping people with new SCIs adjust after rehab. "I used to go to their houses and talk to them about getting back to life," she says. "I'd teach them how to plan a budget, hire PCAs, make meals, and take care of their personal hygiene. I shared my own background to get them going, and I found that the more I talked about my injury, the more it helped them—and the better it made *me* feel."

Tales from the Workplace

Thanks in large part to the assistance of professionals like Purcell—as well as the same determination they used to get through rehab—many of my patients and thousands of others with paralysis have been able to resume working post-injury, either in their own fields or in new professions. For many of them, first-person experience with SCI and an innate desire to help others tackle the challenges that come with it have provided for a satisfying professional fit—as was the case for Cindy Purcell.

Marlene was a paramedic and firefighter for fifteen years before the car accident in which she fractured her tenth thoracic vertebra. Because of her paraplegia, she was unable to do what she loved, which included teaching paramedics at the college level. Some people previously employed in physically demanding jobs like Marlene's have been able to find a way to remain in the same fields after SCI; con-

sider, for example, the paralyzed construction worker who uses his creativity and past onsite experiences to become a general contractor, or the dancer who further develops her talents to become a choreographer. For Marlene, however, this option was too emotionally difficult. "I was in a kind of mourning for the loss of my old life," she recalls. "It was tough seeing my buddies at weddings and other celebrations, where talk always seemed to revolve around what was going on at work. I knew I couldn't go back to that job in a way that would satisfy me, but I still had an urge to help people."

Figuring that it might be her best shot, but not holding out much real hope, Marlene applied online for an advocacy position with her local chapter of the National Spinal Cord Injury Association. "When I had my interview, I told them I couldn't even believe that they had called me back," she remembers with a laugh. "They said a lot of people lose their confidence about working when they get injured, and that made me feel better. Then they gave me the job. Now I'm doing Early Intervention with SCI patients, helping them learn that there is life after injury. I help them find places to live and hook them up with peer and support people. It makes me feel like I'm doing something worthwhile again."

Even those who don't choose to work directly with the SCI community frequently find a way to incorporate into their work lives the insights and sensitivity they have gained through their own experiences. Take Drew, who became an elementary school teacher after a diving accident in his early twenties.

Knowing that the fourth-graders in his first class would be naturally curious about having a teacher with paraplegia, Drew decided to deal with the situation straight on. "The first day, I asked them, 'Raise your hand if you notice I'm in a wheelchair,'" he explains. "Everybody raised their hands, of course, so I said, 'Good. Now I'm not going to tell you about how I got this way for a couple of weeks.

In the meantime, I want you to observe.' I wanted them to be comfortable and familiar enough with me that they would think of the best possible questions. I brought in a poster of pictures showing me doing sports like skiing and skydiving, so they could see some of the things that disabled people are capable of. And by halfway through the year, most of them didn't even see me in a wheelchair anymore.

"I've done the same exercise every year since," Drew continues, "and I always get a great response. I'm teaching third-graders now, and because they get those first few weeks to know me, they don't ask things like, 'How do you eat?' and 'How do you write?' They know all that by then, so they come up with more insightful questions like, 'How do your own kids view you?' or 'How do you feel about not standing for so many years?' I answer as best as I can, telling them about how my kids have never known me not in a wheelchair, and how I can still do a lot of the same things any dad can. I talk about my standing table at home, which I use when I can to help my bones and muscles stay strong. These conversations help the students develop a deeper understanding of the disabled experience, and bring us all closer together."

Thanks to such honest discussion about disability, as well as the increased presence of people with SCI in all areas of life, we are raising a generation that is more tolerant and accepting of people's differences. Long gone are the days when a politician like President Franklin Roosevelt (a polio patient) had to hide from the public his inability to walk unaided. In fact, today many people with SCI have been able to make their mark politically at both the local and the national level, including Sam Sullivan of Vancouver, British Columbia.

After a skiing accident at age nineteen left him with C4-C5 tetraplegia, Sullivan suffered a long bout of depression and was forced to go on welfare for seven years because he couldn't get his life back on track. Then, while dressing one morning, he had an epiphany. Frustrated by the amount of time it took him to get ready, he did a "detailed time-usage analysis" and realized that he could free up six weeks of his life just by putting a sock and shoe on the same foot sequentially rather than putting a sock on each foot first and then moving on to the shoes.

So inspired, the lifelong Vancouver resident realized that there were other things he could do to make his life more efficient, and he went on to design a series of homemade adaptive devices. These included an abdominal belt to support his weakened stomach, a leg bag system that uses suction to cut down on bladder infections, and an extended clothes hanger hook to reach for and pick up items. Further motivated by his success, he later founded an organization, the Tetra Society, through which engineers, mechanics, and other volunteers worked together to make similar innovative gadgets a reality for other disabled people. From these beginnings, Sullivan soon built a group of six non-profit agencies to help people with disabilities around Canada and the world gain easier access to activities like music, sailing, and gardening. (See www.disabilityfoundation.org).

Taking note of Sullivan's charisma and leadership skills, legislators whom he had met encouraged the entrepreneur to run for a position on the Vancouver city council. He did so, won, and after serving for twelve years, pursued the office of mayor in 2005. Despite being an underdog in both the primary and the general elections, he claimed victory and became chief executive of Canada's third-largest city— and the first individual with tetraplegia to head a North American city of any size. Once in office, Sullivan used the same successful, no-nonsense approach that he had taken in establishing his foundation to tackle challenges like drugs and crime. He became known beyond his province when he took part in the closing ceremonies of the 2006 Winter Olympics. Representing Vancouver, which was to be the host city for the Winter Games in 2008, he captivated the *crowd in the Turin stadium and a worldwide television audience by holding the Canadian flag in one hand and moving his wheelchair back and forth to make it wave. Among the fan mail he received after the broadcast was a letter from a fellow wheelchair user in Virginia, who thanked him for bringing "tears to my eyes and a sense of triumph! I truly appreciated the fact that you chose not to have someone wave it for you."*

Another person who knows all too well about not giving up easily is Elmer Bartels. When he was injured in 1960, people with paralysis faced an extra challenge in returning to productive lives: a lack of role models. Even though the average life expectancy rates for SCI patients began climbing in the 1940s and 1950s from just a few weeks post-injury to decades or more, most of the general public and many in the medical field simply didn't expect this growing population to successfully reintegrate into the general workforce or student population. And for a while, owing largely to apathy and inertia, they were right.

"I broke my neck as a senior at Colby College, playing a game of inter-fraternity hockey, and just like that became a quadriplegic," explains Bartels. "Even though I was just twenty-two years old and had the rest of my life in front of me, I was told that I had a limited life expectancy and limited prospects for accomplishments compared with my non-disabled peers. The general thinking then was that you'd go back to your family or to a nursing home and be taken care of for the rest of your life. There was no expectation whatsoever that you could go back to work or school."

Bartels, who came from a supportive family, didn't buy it. During rehab, he met a group of other young men with whom he shared stories and dreams. They've remained close ever since. "We began to teach each other how to really live. Although there were not a lot of

examples of people who had done it before us, we talked about re-
turning to school and going on to careers."

Within a year Bartels was back at Colby, living in accessible quar-
ters at a hotel near campus. His new wife, Mary, who had been one
of his rehab nurses, served as his primary caregiver, and he went on
to graduate from Colby and earn a master's degree in nuclear physics from Tufts University in 1964. The support of his wife, parents,
and professors helped Bartels believe that he could do anything, but
this didn't mean everybody else agreed. "I applied for a job at an op-
tical physics company after getting my master's, and the department head was ready to hire me. They started putting the paper-
work through, but then the company's medical consultant
recommended against hiring me. The offer was quickly taken off the
table. Sure I was pissed off, but I wound up getting a job at MIT
shortly thereafter."

In addition to taking a position with MIT's renowned Laboratory
for Nuclear Science, Bartels became a leader in national efforts to
gain rights for those with spinal cord injury and other physical disabilities. After the Independent Living Movement took hold in California, he was one of the key advocates for developing a similar program in Massachusetts. The establishment of the Boston Center for
Independent Living in 1974, the first such facility in the eastern
United States, offered an alternative to institutionalized living and
enabled disabled people who were unemployed and supported by
Medicaid to qualify for free assistance for personal care attendants.
Eventually Massachusetts passed another initiative that today allows
those who are working to get free PCA coverage as well. Once a person's income passes a certain limit, he or she can continue to receive
the coverage and other medical services by paying a monthly pre-
mium based on total income.

By this time, Bartels was a father of two and had moved on to a
new management position at Honeywell Information Systems. He
continued his work on behalf of the disabled community, however,

and in 1977 then-Massachusetts Governor Michael Dukakis asked him to leave his current job to become commissioner of the Mass. Rehabilitation Commission. Bartels accepted the offer—making him just the second person with a severe disability to head a state reha- bilitation agency—and thirty years later, shortly before his 2007 re- tirement, he was continuing the fight to ensure that almost every disabled person who wants a job can get one. "If someone wants to go to work, the public vocational rehabilitation program can help them do so by providing almost any good or service you can think of," he says. "Work training, assistive technology, adaptive work on their home, a ramp, a van modification, you name it."

Bartels has been a mentor not only to me personally but also to many other professionals, and countless people with disabili- ties have benefited from his efforts. Among them is my former patient Charlie, a young man who broke his neck at age nine- teen in a motorbike accident. After about a year of living at home and adjusting to his condition, Charlie began meeting with a job counselor at the Mass. Rehabilitation Commission (MRC). She told him about a job opening near his home at the national headquarters of a large retail chain; he applied for the position and was granted an interview. The job required handling customer inquiries by phone and tracking them elec- tronically, and his counselor had confidence that Charlie could handle it. After all, he could type faster than most able-bodied people thanks to a makeshift method he had designed himself using two pencils, a bottle cap, a track ball, and a Popsicle stick to compensate for his weakened fingers.

"The interview wasn't hard, because my counselor had told them I was tetraplegic, and she came with me to the meeting," he recalls. "What was tough was when I got the job and found out I was the only person in a building of 3,000 who was in a wheelchair. Obvi-

ously everybody looked at me, and some of them felt obligated to tell me a story about their nephew or someone they knew who was also in a chair. Then there were the people who I could tell were trying not to stare and wouldn't even look me in the eye when they walked right by me. It got me down at first, but after a while I decided I had to get over it and not wallow in self-pity. If I acted confident and friendly, things would get better. And they did. Now I have plenty of friends at work, and some people even fight to see who can get to the elevator quickest to push the 'down' button for me."

No matter what job a person chooses after SCI, however, he or she should be prepared to deal with the occasional stares like Charlie did—or sometimes much worse. Even some people in the medical field (a profession where you might expect the *most* understanding) have shown surprisingly little sensitivity when it comes to colleagues with disabilities. Jerry's story is a perfect example. An honors graduate of medical school, he was completing his residency in anesthesiology at a prominent New England hospital when he crushed his T3 and T4 vertebrae in a racing bike crash. Suddenly some of the same young doctors with whom he had been training became members of his own acute care team, and it didn't take him long to start pondering the long-term ramifications of his paralysis.

"I remember cursing like mad in the hospital," Jerry recalls. "I had always been a very physical guy—playing football and soccer, running track, doing triathlons—and now I felt like that part of my life had been closed off. Being in medicine, I'm sure I already knew in the back of my mind that things weren't looking very good for my chosen career, either. Right after the accident, the department [anesthesia] was very supportive, and since almost everybody knew me at the medical center where I was initially treated, there were always people following me around and encouraging me. Pretty soon I got to thinking, 'Maybe I can do this. Maybe I can still be a doctor.'"

Although Jerry knew that returning to his residency program just four months after his injury would be a huge physical and mental challenge, he found that he could get around fine in his wheelchair and that his academic and interpersonal skills remained strong. The biggest obstacles he faced were not caused by his paraplegia, or at least not directly. Now the problem was how others treated him.

"Some of my supervisors were great, but others seemed to go out of their way to make things difficult for me," he says. "I still had to do the same cases and carry the same load as the other residents, but now they would get on me about every detail or claim I was lazy if I missed some of my rotations because of a urinary tract infection or some other medical problem. You'd think they would be more compassionate and empathic of what I was going through, but all I can assume is that maybe some of them had to struggle so hard to become doctors that they couldn't accept the fact that someone who was physically disabled was capable of doing it, too.

"I eventually switched to a different residency back home in Texas, where things got better, but people still questioned my abilities," he continues. "For example, the first time I was pushing a patient back from the OR to the recovery room, I noticed that there was an attendant walking behind me giving the other docs a thumbs-up. Everybody was wondering whether the paralyzed guy could handle himself, and they quickly found out I could. Most of the patients were okay about having a doctor in a wheelchair, but there was one guy whom I was preparing for surgery who came right out and said something like, 'You should be the one on the stretcher going into the OR.' He apologized later, but I never forgot the feeling."

Jerry became interested in pain management, a sub-specialty of anesthesiology, owing to its complexity as well as the opportunity for him to "be a pioneer" and "fight for the underdog." Yet here, again, he encountered another obstacle: a division head who didn't believe a doctor in a wheelchair could handle the job and only agreed to Jerry's participation on a probationary basis.

Employment interviews were no picnic either, as he relived much

of the same prejudice he had dealt with during his residency train-
ing. "I had scored in the top 2 percent of my in-service exam, had
been chief resident, and had a great-looking resume," he recounts.
"But as soon as I showed up in my wheelchair, nobody wanted to
hire me. One hospital even had a guy walk around with a pedome-
ter calculating how many miles I would need to cover during a
twenty-four-hour call. It was something like five miles, and they told
me that it was too far for me to handle. They also told me they were
sure I couldn't intubate [insert a tube into the trachea or windpipe
of] a person in bed. What they didn't bother to do was actually test
how far I could walk or whether I could intubate somebody."

While it might have been easier and even understandable for Jerry
to give up on medicine and pursue a less-demanding career where
his keen intellect would be an advantage and his abilities would not
be questioned, once again he chose to prove the naysayers wrong.
With the support of his wife, family, and friends, he finished his resi-
dency requirements and took a job in anesthesiology at a small, ru-
ral hospital, where he spent much of his spare time studying pain
management. Today he runs a clinic specializing in that area, and
his patients look to him as somebody with a deep appreciation for
their condition. "My patients aren't glad I'm in a wheelchair," he
says, "but they tell me they think I can understand a lot better what
they're going through."

Stories like Jerry's demonstrate that though things are improving in the workplace for people with SCI, old challenges and
stereotypes still exist. "Unfortunately, the attitude in much of society is still that people with disability can't work," says Elmer
Bartels. "It's getting better, but it's still there. We just finished up
a [2007] study that tells us only 30 percent of people with disabilities aged sixteen to seventy-four are employed, whereas 70 percent of the general, nondisabled population is working. Disability and poverty go together; if you don't work, you're bound to a
life of SSI payments, which are less than $12,000 per year."

Having success stories to point to can help people change their circumstances, and there are certainly no shortage of role models now available to someone pondering a return to work after paralysis. Each year the National Spinal Cord Injury Association (NSCIA) honors several individuals with SCI for their vocational achievements and names others to its "Hall of Fame" for their accomplishments and advocacy efforts. Inductees range from celebrities like singer Teddy Pendergrass and Emmy Award–winning TV journalist John Hockenberry to lesser-known entrepreneurs like Marilyn Hamilton, who, frustrated by her cumbersome fifty-pound wheelchair, designed a lightweight model known as the "Quickie" that the NSCIA has credited with "revolutionalizing the wheelchair industry." In addition to being named California Businesswoman of the Year, she found time to give back further by creating a scouting program for disabled children called WOW (Winners on Wheels).

"We still have a long way to go," says Bartels, "and the only thing that will change peoples' attitudes both in the public and in the medical community is convincing people with disabilities that they *can* go back to work and be better off because of it."

Back to School

In the first several hours after he fell from a high ladder during a landscaping job, Vinnie remembered drifting in and out of consciousness. "I woke up once and saw my brother beside me, holding my arms, and I could hear the ambulance coming. They put me on a stretcher, I passed out, and when I came to I was in the hospital. I thought I had broken my legs, and I couldn't figure out why they hadn't put any casts on them. My English was not strong, so they explained it to my wife and she told me: 'You didn't break your legs, you broke your spine.'

"I just cried and cried. I was thirty-seven and didn't know what was going to happen to me," he explains. "I had come to the United

*States about ten years before from Portugal, where I had dropped
out of school after the fifth grade. Besides landscaping and other
manual labor, there wasn't much I was qualified to do. After I got
out of rehab I needed someone to take me to doctor's appointments
and interpret for me, so my wife would have to come home from
work early and take me at night. She was the only one in the family
with a job, so I hated making her do that. She was always so tired,
and I felt like I wasn't doing anything to help her or my family."*

Vinnie's predicament is a common one for many patients in
the months and years after spinal cord injury. Trained for jobs
that they are no longer physically able to perform, they can feel
helpless and unsure of what to do with themselves. And while
individuals like those described in the previous pages have been
able to make the transition to new positions in or outside their
fields, for others the best solution might be what Vinnie and his
wife decided he would do: go back to school.

Why take this route? Education is a definite advantage for employment no matter what a person's physical abilities, so logic
dictates that if you're not sure what job is best for you—or what
you're best qualified for—taking classes in different areas may
be a great way to both pinpoint your interests and strengths and
make yourself more marketable to future employers. Some people with SCI have even come to view their injury as an impetus
toward finishing high school or pursuing the college degree
they had put off earlier. Research findings support this plan of
action: People with higher education find greater success in
reemployment after paralysis and tend to earn more money than
those with less education.

As with returning to work, of course, there are logistical issues and concerns to consider when going back to school. But
just as the growth of the Independent Living Movement and
the passage of the Americans with Disabilities Act have led to

greater opportunities and less discrimination in the workplace, these and other initiatives have also helped expand educational options for men and women with spinal cord injury. Some disabled people fear that inaccessible classrooms and dormitories might be a major obstacle, but under the provisions of the Rehabilitation Act of 1973, any secondary school or college that receives federal funding is required to make its academic and living facilities wheelchair accessible. Furthermore, many colleges and universities now have an Office for Students with Disabilities (or the equivalent) charged with maximizing the educational opportunities for such individuals. These facilities can provide staff assistance for note taking, access to computers and personal attendants, and a variety of other services.

For a certain segment of the SCI population, going back to school is about more than just future employment; for the large number of individuals who are injured in their late teens and early twenties, it's also about reuniting with their peer group. Many of my patients are young men and women who were in college or just about to start when they were injured, and thus they later faced the challenge of returning to campus in a wheelchair.

"I was so depressed when I first went back to school," says Danny, who was a freshman at a major eastern university when a car accident left him with paraplegia. "There were many days of frustration and emotional turmoil. It hit me like a ton of bricks. Here I am with all these able-bodied students, and I can't partake of the same things as them. I was trying to deal with my disability and all the regular pressures of being a freshman at the same time."

Working with the school's office for disabled students, Danny and his family arranged to have a PCA come to his dorm room each morning. "He helped me stretch my legs, take a shower, get some food, and get dressed and out the door. They had a program where you could have somebody go around with you all day helping you get to class and taking notes, but I figured if I was on my own and needed help, I'd ask for it—and that's how I would meet people. It worked great; people were willing to help and I started getting over my anxiety."

Danny still had frustrations, like dealing with snow, ice, frigid temperatures, and huge hills on the way to class or the occasional bowel accident once he got there. But the confidence he gained getting around on his own helped him through the tough times. Although he lived alone as a freshman, he had roommates for three out of five years and made friends all over campus. *"I didn't rush a fraternity, because I didn't want special privileges as a pledge. I got to be friendly with a lot of the guys in one house, and eventually they made me an honorary brother. They invited me to all their parties and formals, and I could tell it was genuine. They loved throwing me around the couch and popping wheelies in my chair, just like they ragged on each other in different ways."*

Danny also made a point of getting to know other disabled people on campus as well as members of the administration to whom he could turn with problems or suggestions. *"It got to the point where I became an advocate for myself—and for others,"* he says. *"I could go into the administrator's office and say, 'Look, I was just like you, I could walk. Now I can't, and it could happen to you in a second. How would you feel if there was no electronic door on a certain building and you couldn't get it open to go to class?'"*

After experiencing spinal cord injury and rehab, some returning students may have a new outlook. Drew, the teacher introduced earlier in this chapter, had been a nineteen-year-old sophomore at a large West Coast university before his injury. Like many undergrads, he was unsure of what he wanted to do with his life. He tried majoring in finance, then psychology, but neither excited him. Only after his injury did Drew find something that truly satisfied him: talking with newly hospitalized SCI patients about his own post-rehab experiences. Very soon, this led to another opportunity—and a career.

"The therapists saw how much I enjoyed it, and how much it helped me grow as a person and deal with my own injury, so they asked me if I wanted to get involved with a trauma prevention program," he recalls. "They had me go to elementary and high schools and talk to kids about being safe—wearing their helmets when they skateboarded or biked, diving feet first into pools the first time, things like that. When the physical and occupational therapists who went with me made their presentations, the kids in the audience would all be talking to each other. But when I went on in my wheelchair, everybody got real quiet. The kids listened to me; I think I hit them right where it counted. I'd go home on a real high about it, and so my father said to me, 'Why don't you go into teaching?' For once I listened to him, and I've never regretted it."

The high cost of a college education need not deter aspiring disabled students, either, as many State Vocational Departments offer financial assistance for tuition, supplies, and other expenses. For those whose spinal cord injury or related medical conditions *do* prevent them from physically attending class some or all of the time, a variety of Internet-based GED and college courses (and even entire undergraduate degrees) are available to anybody with computer access.

Vocational rehab counselor Cindy Purcell, who has advised many others with SCI about returning to work or school, will never forget her own first day of college, which came a few years after her injury.

"I was really nervous, and as my electric wheelchair hummed while rolling down the corridors, I felt like everybody was looking up and

staring at me. For my first class I decided I would try to stay near the back of the room to blend in, but as I was moving down the aisle I was suddenly blocked by a pregnant woman whose legs were sticking out from her desk. I said 'Excuse me' but she didn't respond. I said it again, and then a third time, but still nothing. Finally, the guy next to her tapped her on the shoulder and said, 'Can you please move so she can get by?' The woman looked up at me, rolled her eyes, and then finally shifted herself so I could get past her and to a desk. 'This is some great first day of school,' I thought.

"Needless to say, I was feeling pretty crappy, but within five minutes the same guy who got the woman to move asked if I needed anything. That made me feel better. The next class, he came up to me and said, 'I noticed you were having trouble taking notes, so I made a copy of mine for you.' He wound up helping me with notes the whole semester, because it was hard for me to write with the splint that holds my pencil or pen. My professor also let me take all my tests orally, and a guy in the maintenance office even rigged the elevator I used to get to class so I could open it with a garage door opener instead of using a key.

"So school ended up being a lot like everything else you deal with after injury. Some people you come across will always be fearful of the unknown, like disability, and ignore you or act badly, but then there will be others who couldn't be nicer. You just have to learn not to let the first group bother you."

Back to Play

Steve was sixteen years old when he fell from a tree in his backyard while recovering a football, resulting in T10-T11 paraplegia. A high school swimmer and a baseball and basketball player before his injury, he credits sports with aiding his mental rehabilitation. "I was an angry guy when I got hurt, and I had a real chip on my shoulder

*until I got back into sports," he admits. "Sports gave me an outlet
for my energy and gave me confidence that I could be 'me' again. I
especially liked wheelchair basketball because I could do it with able-
bodied people as well as other guys in chairs. The challenge of getting to the basket and dealing with guys cutting in front of me
helped me learn how to get around in general, and playing on a
team got me going again socially. I became self-confident to the
point where when I went back to college, I was taking on guys from
the school team in HORSE [a shooting game]—and beating them."*

*An engineer by trade, Steve eventually made a second career out
of helping to improve athletic opportunities for the disabled community. Head of a regional wheelchair basketball organization for several years, he's also helped teach kids with SCI and other injuries
how to ski and play other sports. "As a mentor, it's not just seeing
you ski that impacts these kids, but also just how you get in and out
of your car, up to the mountain, and around on your chair. I have a
son whose friend has spina bifida and didn't think disabled people
could swim. Then he saw me jump in, and by the end of the week-
end he was swimming."*

As with work and school, sports and other leisure pursuits
provide some of the best ways to adjust to lifestyle changes
caused by spinal cord injury. Those of my patients who remain
active in this way after discharge from rehab report better overall health, less depression and anxiety, and a greater sense of
personal fulfillment. In fact, studies show a close link between
recreation and employment: Participating in sports builds confidence and teaches cooperation and teamwork—all beneficial
qualities in the workplace. Steve cites his own sports experiences as a big factor in his successful adaptation to life in a
wheelchair, whether at school, on the court, or in the workplace.

Starting in inpatient rehabilitation, a recreational therapist
can be instrumental in helping a newly paralyzed individual find

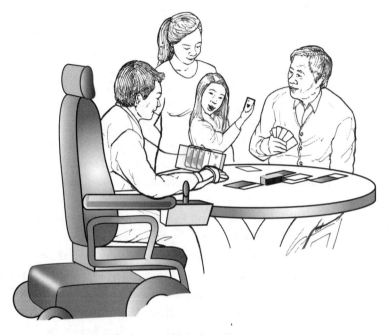

FIGURE 4.   Getting dealt a good hand and keeping it to oneself is still possible for those with limited grasp or hand function, thanks to adaptive equipment like this card holder.

his "recreational niche." As with vocational rehab, the essential ingredients for an effective recreational therapy program include assessment, education, and skill building. Areas of focus range from indoor activities such as painting and other arts and crafts to various wheelchair sports and outdoor recreation like horseback riding, fishing, rock climbing, and sailing. Activities like these are a vital part of living for all people, including those with disabilities. Besides being enjoyable, they help improve a person's self-image and physical well being, while providing an opportunity to meet others and feel connected (see Figure 4).

For some people with SCI, leisure pursuits are a form of self-expression and release, a way to control stress and anxiety. Participating in athletics and competitive pastimes provides a sense of accomplishment and meaning. By "playing," they feel that they can continue to lead healthy, productive, and happy lives. And with the right amount of interest and motivation, almost any recreational activity can be adapted for those who are paralyzed.

One of the first major sports to become popular in the SCI community was wheelchair basketball. Introduced after World War II to former servicemen who were wheelchair dependent yet still possessed the energy of young men in their twenties and thirties, the sport has grown to include men, women, and children of all abilities. Today there are more than 175 teams in the National Wheelchair Basketball Association (or NWBA). The game's appeal is multifaceted: courts are easy to move across on wheels, the ball is big enough so that even people without much finger strength can handle it, and the sense of teamwork, camaraderie, and competitiveness the games promote invigorates those who play. Over time, as athletes at all levels have become more serious about the sport, people like Steve have begun seeking—and in some cases designing themselves—lighter, more durable, and faster wheelchairs to play in. This kind of ingenuity is not limited to basketball, either; one man whose son had a congenital defect of the spine decided to design a custom-built sports wheelchair when he saw his son struggling to move across their back lawn in his standard wheelchair. His model, known as the "Action Chair," has become an important all-terrain vehicle.

Many opportunities exist for disabled athletes today. Virtually every team and individual sport imaginable is being played by paralyzed men, women, and kids with the help of adaptive equipment and standard or specialized wheelchairs: soccer, softball, racquetball, tennis, even scuba diving and rock climbing. There are aerobics instructors with SCI ("sit and be fit" is a pop-

ular mantra), "sled hockey" players who glide over the ice in contraptions that look like souped-up flexible flyers, golfers who hit
the links in specialized carts operated by hand controls, and
even disabled race car drivers. Skiers tackle tough slopes in a variety of devices such as the mono-ski, a molded bucket seat on a
metal frame with a suspension system attached to a single ski.
Because all ski resorts in the United States are now required to
provide equal opportunities to all visitors in compliance with the
ADA, skiing has become a particularly popular pastime for individuals with spinal cord injuries. As one mono-skier explained:
"It's the most amazing opportunity to find out how capable I am.
I feel capable, strong, and free when I'm on the mountain."

The success and growth of disabled sports are due in large
part to the exposure given to them every four years in the Paralympic Games, which are held three weeks after each Winter
and Summer Olympics in the same host cities. More than 3,800
athletes from 136 countries competed in the Athens Paralympic
Games of 2004, squaring off in events from track and field
and swimming to powerlifting and judo. Now the second-largest
sports competition in the world (after the Olympics), the Para-
lympics have several divisions of athletes, including amputees,
those with cerebral palsy, and those in wheelchairs, including
people with spinal cord injuries (see Figure 5).

Wheelchair road racing is another area that has grown significantly in recent years, with top performers like wheelchair
marathoners Jean Driscoll and Jim Knaub becoming well known
among many sports fans, even outside the disabled community.
Whereas they once competed and finished anonymously, wheelchair racers like these are now breaking the tape and collecting trophies and prize money, just like their able-bodied counterparts. Uplifting stories of the determination these athletes
display in reaching the top are commonly found in disability
magazines, on websites, and in the mainstream press. Some top

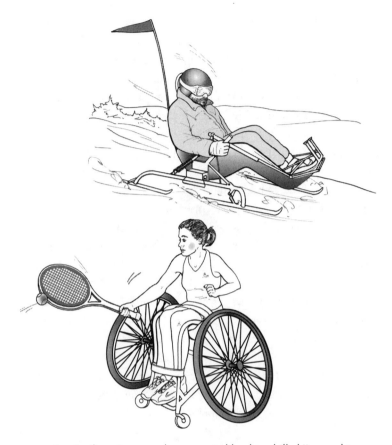

FIGURE 5.   As these images show, sports like downhill skiing and tennis are still open to athletes after spinal cord injury.

performers have even earned commercial endorsements: Paralympic track and field champ Doug Heir, who has collected more than 200 gold medals in national and international competition, has joined the ranks of Michael Jordan and Tiger Woods in having his face on a Wheaties box.

Most Paralympic sports are also available to people with SCI at the amateur level. In recent years, quad rugby has become a popular option for athletes who like things a bit more physical. The popular documentary film *Murderball*, released in 2005, introduced audiences worldwide to this intense sport, in which men with tetraplegia who still maintain some arm movement play a full-contact version of the game (a hybrid of American football and soccer). The rules include passing a ball up the court toward a goal, much like wheelchair basketball, except here players can slam their specially constructed chairs into opponents and even topple them over to regain possession of the ball. Many of the young men on the top-ranked United States quad rugby team have spinal cord injuries, and the Oscar-nominated movie reveals the physical, emotional, and social challenges they faced post-injury on their path to the 2004 Paralympic Games in Atlanta.

"The first allure was always the contact," Mark Zupan, captain of the 2004 U.S. quad rugby squad, said in the film of what drew him to the sport after he broke his neck in a car accident. "Where else can you hit somebody as hard as you possibly want to or can in a chair? . . . I played college soccer before I was hurt, and just to be able to jump back into something that you could be so competitive at or you can achieve . . . it's unreal."

A civil engineer by training, Zupan became a motivational speaker and an author after the film's release and was pleased that the documentary helped dispel many of the myths about athletes in wheelchairs. Many people with SCI (like him) can indeed feel pain in their legs, and even if they can't, they still have ways to tell if something's wrong. For instance, sweating above the level of injury or involuntary movements of a foot or leg could be a sign of dysreflexia (an uncontrolled increase in blood pressure unique to spinal cord injuries at the level of T5 or above that occurs as a result of a noxious stimulus) or an indication of a broken bone or another serious injury, respectively. (See Chapter 11.)

Traditionally competitive sports, of course, are not the only pastimes that can be enjoyed after injury. Ted Purcell likes to go fly-fishing with his son, Tanner, and he doesn't let his C7 spinal cord injury keep him away from the water. Billiards and bowling are also popular among the disabled, and several ingenious devices have been designed to help deliver the biggest, heaviest balls smoothly down a lane. Hunters use all-terrain wheelchairs, and people with SCI regularly take to the water as boaters and wind surfers, and to the sky as pilots, thanks to their determination and adaptive equipment.

As the world has become more accepting of wheelchairs and those in them, pastimes once thought off-limits are now available after injury. Individuals with SCI are now gracing stages, televisions, and movie screens as actors and dancers, and some are also going behind the curtain and camera as directors and choreographers. Travel—another area once largely closed off to the disabled—is now possible thanks to dramatically improved wheelchair accessibility in airports and communities around the world. Travel groups have sprung up for wheelchair users, as have many guides describing the "ins and outs" of different cities and countries from a seated perspective. (For a partial listing of sports and travel options, see the Resources section at the back of the book.)

In short, there are currently more opportunities than ever for people to spend their leisure time after paralysis. And though some hobbies may become more difficult after SCI, with a little creativity and determination, you can still participate in the activities you love.

Travis Roy became a famous figure overnight when he slammed into the boards eleven seconds into his first shift on the Boston University

men's hockey team and emerged from the incident with C4-C5
tetraplegia and minimal movement in only one arm. His dreams of
a professional athletic career now shattered, he focused first on fin-
ishing his degree from BU and then on making a living as a motiva-
tional speaker and advocate for the disabled community. He
cowrote a book on his post-injury experiences—titled, appropriately,
"Eleven Seconds"—and started doing a little college hockey broad-
casting. Roy even returned to his old hobby of landscape painting,
with a slight twist: he now held the brush in his mouth.

"I'm a far better painter than I was before," he said in an inter-
view. "When I painted with my hand, I always wanted perfect
straight lines . . . When you paint with your mouth, there's no such
thing as a straight line. There aren't any straight lines in nature."
Roy said it takes him ten to twelve hours over three or four sessions
to create a single work, but the effort is worth it. "A lot of the things
I enjoyed have been taken away from me," he explained. "So the
things I really enjoy, I do on a regular basis."

Success at Last

Eventually, after completing rehab and becoming more experienced with the challenges of spinal cord injury, many of my patients have told me that their paralysis slowly becomes incorpo-
rated into their sense of self. No longer do they feel the need to
hide their disability; nor do they spend each night dreaming that
they will be "back to normal" when they awake. In reaching this
point, they have learned to cope with the physical changes of spinal cord injury and have attained a sense of peace. They now
know how to be their own advocates. They understand when and
how to take responsibility for themselves and, just as significantly, when to seek assistance. This realization has forced some
of them to reevaluate their sense of meaning and purpose.
Moreover, many of my patients have found that the less time

they spend dwelling on their losses, the more likely they are to take advantage of available resources, make necessary accommodations for disability, and ultimately return to an enriching life.

In fact, many people with spinal cord injury have told me that their disability has actually *enhanced* their lives. By learning flexibility and patience, as well as how to manage adversity, they have become more sensitive and accepting of others. Some have even recognized that their injury has been a positive motivating force, pulling them away from a past existence that might have been marked by underachievement, isolation, or even drugs and violence. By confronting the challenges of disability, they have gained a unique confidence that many will never have the opportunity to experience. They've been able to shift their attitudes and goals to recognize that life with paralysis can be happy and productive. These are the people who can ultimately see their disability as just another aspect of life, not the major focus and obstacle of every day. And this, in the end, is the truest sign of successful adjustment.

Dating after SCI: Out and About

Lisa could tell that something had changed the first time her boy-friend visited her in rehab after she broke her neck in a car accident. He ignored her attempts to discuss their future, and he started com-ing to the hospital less and less often. Eventually he broke things off completely. "He never came right out and said it was because of my injury," she recalls, "but he didn't have to—it was obvious to me."

One afternoon a few months later, twenty-six-year-old Lisa was on a community outing with the other spinal cord patients from her unit. "I was seated next to a really outgoing guy named Joe who had paraplegia. He was cute, and I had a great time talking to him, but I just couldn't imagine myself ever being attracted to a guy in a wheelchair," she says with a laugh. "It sounds silly considering I was in one myself, but it's just where I was at the time. I didn't want to be reminded of what had happened to me. But the more I got to know Joe around the unit, the more I liked him. He was flirting with me, even though I almost never had makeup on and looked terrible. For the first time since my injury, I was starting to feel attractive."

After they were discharged from rehab, Lisa and Joe remained in touch by phone and eventually decided to get together. During their first dinner date, the chemistry between them grew stronger as the night went on. It was obvious they both wanted to take the relation-ship to a more physical level, but unspoken concerns remained in the way. Lisa felt self-conscious about her tetraplegia and her need for attendants to help her get around, not to mention her indwelling catheter. Joe, by contrast, was quite comfortable with the possibility

of becoming intimate. Since only his legs were paralyzed, he was far
more independent.

"I was pretty close with my nighttime attendant, Nancy, so I de-
cided to talk it over with her," says Lisa. "I asked her flat out if she
would be comfortable helping me out during an intimate evening if
the opportunity arose down the road. She was very cool about it and
said sure. So when Joe and I decided to go back to my place after
our third or fourth date, Nancy was there to help me get undressed,
put on a new nightgown, and transfer to bed while he waited. Then,
when Joe came in, she quietly left the room."

Most people desire some degree of intimacy and companionship, and a spinal cord injury does not change these basic
wishes. People who are newly injured still dream of finding the
right person to love and to love them. In fact, one of the most
common questions patients have asked me is, "Can I still do it?"
What they usually mean is, "Will I be attractive to anyone? Will I
be able to have sex?"

Many people assume that sexual activity is physically impossible for those with SCI, but this is not the case at all (as will be detailed in Chapter 6). As for relationships, when a couple genuinely wants to be together, it makes little difference whether one
or both partners can walk or fully use their arms. No matter how
serious an injury, the ability to fall in love remains unchanged.
The things that should truly matter in a genuine romantic relationship—mutual attraction, commitment, trust—remain unaf-
fected by paralysis. In Chapter 7 we discuss some keys to making such relationships work and last, but here we focus on the
first steps toward getting out and meeting people.

Back in the Mix

No one can deny, of course, that dating after a spinal cord injury
is different. A person's physical appearance has changed, and

despite greater awareness and sensitivity about wheelchairs than ever before, it's only natural that others may perceive and react differently to someone who uses one. Nonetheless, most people with SCI are apprehensive about dating again, not because they're afraid of how others will judge them, but because they feel inadequate. Some newly injured people have a hard time rebuilding their confidence when they're always having to ask for help. Others wonder why anyone would want to date a person in a wheelchair given the challenges that accompany SCI. Patients have even told me that they feel like the outside world no longer views them as sexual beings capable of romance and intimacy. They have grown tired, they say, of constantly being thought of as just "friends"—never as potential lovers.

Wheel Appeal

The singles scene, with its emphasis on physical appearance, can be frustrating, especially for disabled women. Many men have been socially conditioned to pursue only "perfect" women, which of course eliminates any possibility that they could also be paralyzed. And in a society in which looks can be a crucial factor in making a good first impression, having a spinal cord injury may subsequently be considered a major liability. For example, if a potential partner can get past the metallic rods and rubber wheels, there are the weakened muscles, weight gain or loss, and, in tetraplegia, curled fingers and hands to contend with. Being in a wheelchair can also hamper some of the natural body language so often used to move an initial social encounter forward—like brushing an arm or placing one's feet on the leg of a neighbor's barstool. Increased eye contact and wide, expressive smiles, two methods that people with SCI use to nonverbally convey their interest, may or may not have the desired effect.

There are other times, in contrast, when people regard their wheelchairs as an advantage in social settings. They can be the perfect ice-breaker between strangers, the start of a conversation when someone is curious about why one is needed or when the person in the chair requests or is offered assistance. A few of my patients have admitted that they feel their wheelchairs make them *more* approachable, since the seated position can be less physically intimidating to an interested stranger. Moreover, some able-bodied individuals regard paralyzed people as even more desirable lovers and partners because they presume that their experiences have resulted in heightened emotional sensitivity and inner strength.

Hooking Up

When it comes to deciding whom they want to date, both disabled people and their non-injured counterparts consider many factors. Some able-bodied individuals, for example, always have to be the ones cared for in a relationship. They prefer their partner to be a nurturer rather than someone who needs care, now or in the future. Since these are usually the same people who would never consider asking out a person in a wheelchair, the chances are low that someone with SCI would have to deal with them, anyway.

Other people, however, may develop more subtle concerns after an initial positive encounter with a disabled person. They may fear the public's discrimination or stares, or they might not want to deal with some of the logistical hassles that go along with dating someone who is paralyzed. The need to check ahead and dine only in accessible restaurants, for instance, or to go only to movie theaters with specially designated seats may be too big of an inconvenience for them. The loss of privacy that results when a personal care attendant has to come along on what is supposed to be a romantic dinner for two can also be extremely difficult, even if that attendant is as sensitive and helpful as Lisa's nighttime PCA, Nancy.

Given how little most people know about disability, it's not surprising that some individuals in wheelchairs shy away from dating anyone able-bodied, choosing instead to stay in "their own world." They may make this choice out of concern that those seeking relationships with them are only looking to satisfy a personal need or to have someone depend on them. Understandably, they worry that these able-bodied people may consciously or unconsciously desire to be caregivers rather than share in a mutual relationship, or that they will take off before making a more serious commitment. Yet another worry is the possibility of getting involved with a person who may simply be curious about how it feels to be intimate with someone in a wheelchair.

These fears aside, some people with SCI will choose to date only others in wheelchairs because of the mutual understanding and increased camaraderie they gain from sharing the secrets and frustrations of disability. Asked why they chose to be part of a "double disability" couple, several individuals we spoke with cited the added sensitivity and empathy of those who have faced the daily obstacles of getting along in an able-bodied world. Yet despite such natural bonds, double disability couples also experience their own unique set of challenges. More specifically, each partner must learn about and get used to the other's limitations, especially when the disabilities are different. Sometimes the challenges can be particularly intense, as when two aides are required to help with positioning during intimate moments.

On the other hand, many paralyzed individuals assert that they would *never* date another person in a wheelchair. This group may be concerned that outsiders would always assume that it is only disability holding them together, not a genuine relationship. This kind of attitude, though, could really be a reflection of the person's own insecurities, or his or her fear of the additional attention that being part of such a twosome might create. For these people, dealing with their own specific disability issues is enough; "double" discrimination or social stigma may be too much to imagine. As a result, they stick to relationships involving people free of disability.

In the end, we should not judge a person's decision either to exclusively date other people with disabilities or to date only the able-bodied. What matters is the meaning behind the choice. After all, most people in successful relationships come to realize that their selection of a significant other actually has more to do with shared values, genuine affection, and mutual commitment than with their or their partner's ability to walk.

Presenting One's Disability

"After I got hurt, I was worried that I would never have another girl-friend or get married—I'd never have somebody to share my life with," says Charlie, a young man with C4-C5 tetraplegia who was hurt in a motorbike accident when he was nineteen. "My whole day was scheduled, so I couldn't be as free as I wanted. I needed an aide who could stay over after I was put to bed in case I wanted a girl to come by. I couldn't move in bed, so it was difficult to have sex, but you find ways to compensate. It's intimidating at first for a girl, but I figured if somebody couldn't deal with it, she wasn't going to be right."

No matter what the social situation, people with disabilities like spinal cord injury can benefit from a unique interpersonal skill—the capacity to "contain" their disability. As noted by the psychologist Rhoda Olkin, author of *What Psychotherapists Should Know about Disability*, this means being able to have others look past their appearance to see what they really have to offer. Say, for example, a disabled person notices that others seem uncomfortable around his wheelchair. The more he can make them feel at ease and focus on the actual person sitting before them, the greater the chances that the chair will become less of a focus. The success of this ability depends on the paralyzed person's own comfort level with his or her injury. Other people's anxieties are more likely to subside when an individual is at ease with the circumstances, no matter how limited his or her functioning. The key is becoming skilled at presenting one's disability openly and without judgment, so that it never becomes an awkward or intimidating intrusion when meeting others.

Although being paralyzed can dramatically alter how a person sees himself (as discussed in Chapters 2 and 3), he can eventually establish a new and healthy identity with the right amount of effort. By going back to work, resuming one's role as a stay-at-home parent, or successfully completing rehab and returning to independent living, an individual can learn to appreciate his inner spirit and abilities. Many of my patients have found it easier to be open and reveal their positive qualities to others after realizing that they still have much to offer post-injury. Once a person rediscovers passion and optimism, expressed through words, thoughts, and actions, the interest of others will deepen, enabling them to look past any obvious physical differences. To be sure, this is a long and difficult process for many people with SCI. But in my practice I've met many individuals whose confidence and belief in their own worth have allowed them to take more social risks; as a result, others have seen past their disability.

Take the experiences of Danny, the eighteen-year-old who was paralyzed just before his freshman year of college. His story demonstrates how a person can use this type of confidence to rebound from negative experiences and create positive ones. Danny's problem wasn't meeting girls; it was getting them to take him seriously as a guy, rather than as a guy in a wheelchair.

"The dynamic of going into a bar and meeting women or talking to a girl at a fraternity party wasn't really the place for somebody with a disability to thrive," he recalls. "Even though I was in the bars and at the parties, it was tough. Let's face it, men and women go to those places for one reason—to hook up. I'm not saying I didn't have fun, but it was the same scenario all the time. I'd have a gorgeous girl on my lap and she'd whisper to me: 'If only you could walk, I'd be your girlfriend.' You know how many times I got that? Or a gorgeous girl was sitting on my lap kissing me, and the next thing I knew I was wheeling myself home alone at the end of the night while she was walking the other way with her able-bodied boyfriend. I was like some kind of doll or something."

Danny managed to get through this period by learning not to feel sorry for himself. "You just need to turn things around," he says, "and only by getting to really know people and forming friendships that may bloom into more can you help yourself and others see past the wheelchair and its awkward unknowns.

"When I was on campus, away from the bar scene, and I got to meet women in a different type of setting—that was my playing field," he adds. "Most of my success was in the student center and the library. I always looked for that pretty girl behind the book. There I didn't have to worry about beer or fraternity guys. It was just me; I was on my own court. I would wait for a girl to come in, then I would say, 'Can you help me?' She'd say, 'Sure, what do you need?' and this would give me the opportunity to introduce myself and ask all about her as she helped me grab a book on a high shelf. That's how I made a lot of my friends. They would see me later on campus and come up and say hi. The next thing I knew I was eating at sorority houses all the time."

Some people who have been unable to develop this kind of positive attitude may instead try to deny their disability and even cover it up. Unfortunately, this approach frequently backfires. Although choosing to walk with crutches rather than using a wheelchair may make a person *think* he or she appears less disabled, the awkward gait or falls that may result can actually draw *more* attention than a wheelchair. The same goes for the person who avoids wearing hand splints in restaurants and winds up with a lap full of food. Others may, in fact, become even more uncomfortable around people who seem to be trying too hard to downplay their paralysis.

A person's ease with his or her own body is another important factor in attracting the interest of others. After a spinal cord injury, many people become understandably sensitive about changes in their appearance. Our society places a great deal of importance on physical attributes; from movies and television to billboards and magazine ads, the "ideal look" is everywhere. Yet compared to this standard of perfection, almost *any* person would come up lacking. And for someone with a spinal cord injury, using such a model to measure oneself against can only damage self-esteem. With some notable exceptions in recent years, including actor/activist Christopher Reeve, TV newsman John Hockenberry, and singer Teddy Pendergrass, people in wheelchairs have been largely absent from the mainstream media and pop culture.

Yet with time and experience, a person with SCI can learn to keep outside biases in perspective and adjust to a new body image. A period of deep grief, avoidance of social events, and even depression may ensue beforehand, but eventually the majority of people with spinal cord injuries *do* come to acknowledge and accept their new physical appearance. When this happens, the focus shifts to the positive, and these individuals become more concerned with improving how they look. Many start making the effort to dress more attractively when meeting others for the first time, or choose unique jewelry and flattering hairstyles to

help deflect attention from their wheelchairs. Meticulous grooming also adds to an individual's allure and social charm, as do
strong and confident posture, facial expressions, and body language. And when a person is genuinely able to feel beautiful
again, whether disabled or not, he or she will *act* it. This, in turn,
will undoubtedly increase the likelihood that others will see them
in the same light.

Because there are always people who hesitate before ap-
proaching someone who is paralyzed, patients have told me that
they often feel the need to make the first move when meeting
new people. This kind of outgoing demeanor and comfort with
strangers allows others to recognize that despite their use of mobility aides, people with SCI have much to offer a relationship.
Similarly, many people have found that a sense of humor can
be very valuable. A little laughter will put most people at ease,
especially when dealing with the potentially embarrassing situations that everybody with disabilities dreads—like falling out of
a wheelchair or experiencing bowel or bladder mishaps. In the
long run, people with spinal cord injury want the same thing as
everyone else: partners and friends who can fully accept them
for who they are. Only then does *any* relationship have the best
chance for success.

Getting Out There

Finding romance in the twenty-first century takes some effort.
One thing is for sure: To meet people, an individual must "get
out there" and prevent his or her disability from becoming a lim-
itation. Potential companions can be found almost anywhere—
at restaurants, places of worship, bus stops, work, school, online, even at the grocery store. Opportunities for socializing exist
in exactly the same places as they did *before* spinal cord injury.
The only location anyone can be sure to have little luck meeting

someone special is at home alone . . . and offline. Accordingly, paralyzed people should try to get back into the community as soon as possible post-injury, even if this just means a trip to the neighborhood store. In fact, familiar territory like this can be just the right place for the disabled to experiment with talking about themselves and their new lives. Using this friendly, safe environment to learn how to approach strangers can be quite helpful for someone who is new to a wheelchair. Some people also find it helpful to role play different social situations with close friends and family.

The bottom line is that the more activities you participate in— including volunteer work, religious groups, or community education classes—the more opportunities you have to get to know others socially. Some people may choose to become involved with their local Independent Living Centers or the National Spinal Cord Injury Association (see Resources) to develop a social network. Several couples I know have actually found romance in the hospital setting. Doctors, nurses, and therapists, with their experience and knowledge, are certainly capable of looking past a wheelchair and will also be less likely to feel intimidated or put off by disability. Indeed, many such unions have occurred— albeit after rehabilitation is over!

For those who continue to experience difficulty finding other single people, or who tend to be shy or introverted, dating services and single groups—including those designed specifically for individuals with disabilities—are available. When transportation or physical restrictions are an issue, some may turn to personal ads or online dating services and chat rooms. These venues offer the opportunity to ease back into self-acceptance and intimacy, since no one is disabled in cyberspace or the classifieds unless they want to be. When conversing with others by phone or the computer, people with SCI can relax and not worry about their wheelchairs. Some even purposely delay mentioning their injury because they prefer to "meet" people without worrying that their disability will get in the way. Others, in contrast, have chosen to reveal their use of a wheelchair from the very start. And for individuals who not only want to share such information but are seeking companions in a similar situation, there are websites geared specifically to the disabled dating community.

The most important thing to remember is this: Despite the relationship concerns of those with spinal cord injuries, there *are* still plenty of people who can put physical abilities aside when seeking someone to date. These individuals are able to recognize that the most desirable qualities are intangibles like warmth, honesty, and intelligence. By looking beyond any preconceived notions of what they had always imagined their "perfect" partner would be, they are able to maximize their chance of finding a soul mate, wheelchair or not.

"For the first couple years after my accident, my dating experiences ran the gamut from disappointing to infuriating," recalls Laurie, an attractive lawyer in her thirties who sustained C6 paraplegia as the result of a horseback riding accident. "The few guys I met on blind dates seemed to take one look at me and the next at their watch, while in bars some guys might show real interest, but then wind up spending the night asking me questions about what I could and couldn't do since my injury—not what music, food, or books I liked. The few times that the night went real well and I got intimate with someone, more often than not he wouldn't call me again. To me these felt like the ultimate 'pity dates'—it's as if the guys were hooking up with me just to say they had done their part to help disabled people. Of course, maybe they did this with able-bodied girls, too, but I tended to think the worst.

"Finally, I came up with an idea that I thought might weed out some of the bad ones right off the bat. I joined an online dating ser-

vice and wrote up a profile about myself. I've done personal ads a couple times in the past but never mentioned my injury. This time I added stuff about some of my humorous experiences getting around in a wheelchair, like going to the bank and supermarket. I started the ad 'SWF, 27, seeks someone to help pick my melons,' and got a bunch of responses. A few turned out to be from sensitive, intelligent guys, and when we went out I never got the feeling they were there for any reason other than genuine interest. By not feeling sorry for myself and putting it all out there, I found what I was looking for—people who didn't feel sorry for me either."

In the end, no matter the ultimate rewards of a mutual and fulfilling relationship, the path to getting there may be filled with frustrations and disappointments. The key is to maintain confidence, learn from experience, and continue to persevere. Finding a romantic partner is a challenge for everyone, not only for those who are paralyzed.

6

Sexual Function after SCI:
The Next Challenge

In the two months since the water-skiing accident in which Sarah broke her T10 vertebra, her husband, Mike, had visited her every day in the rehab hospital. One afternoon, when therapy was over and they were alone in her room, he closed the door and curled up into bed next to her, kissing her gently. He expressed interest in exploring further, but Sarah was afraid of the potential disappointment if they tried and "failed." This happened a few more times until one night, without any discussion, Mike began caressing her in a familiar way.

"Even though I couldn't feel anything below my belly button, a huge rush of pleasure came over me," Sarah recalled later. "It wasn't sex like we used to have, but it was still more satisfying than I ever thought it could be again. It was a breakthrough for us as a couple and a big step in my recovery after injury."

Human sexuality is complicated; it encompasses not only sexual drive and desire, interpersonal relations and intimacy, self-understanding and body image, but also sexual function and behaviors. For many in the general public, the possibility that disabled people might have sex seems unimaginable. As a result of this lack of knowledge, paralyzed individuals are often assumed to be non-sexual. Yet while a spinal cord injury does psychologically and physically affect a person's sexuality, it does not end it. Sexual expression is a natural and vital part of human life, whether or not a person can walk. Despite the changes in physical function, the emotional aspects of sexuality continue to be as important for disabled people as for anybody else. As I've seen in my own patients who have resumed physically intimate relationships, being sexual after SCI allows people to feel "whole" again and subsequently improves their overall quality of life.

In technical terms, spinal cord injury affects sexual ability as a result of the physiological changes caused by damage to particular nerve pathways. This may mean diminished genital sensation, loss of adequate erections or the ability to ejaculate for men, and decreased lubrication in women. In addition, decreased muscle strength and involuntary spasms may affect a person's positioning and movement during sexual activity. Depending on the extent and location of the neurological damage, sexual function will vary.

Yet no matter the level of paralysis, all people with SCI will be capable of feeling physical attraction, excitement, desire, and love. They remain just as "sexual" as anyone else, maintaining the potential for intimacy and romantic fulfillment. Sexuality is not only the pleasurable release of orgasm but also a means of communication, and a way to develop and maintain togetherness with another human being. This ability is not lost after injury. As with so many other elements of disability, adjusting to the changes in sexuality is a matter of learning and adaptation.

The alterations in bodily sensations can be shocking at first. Patients have often asked me how sexual activity can be pleasurable when even a tickle or a soft caress can now barely be felt—if at all. Some individuals have become so put off by these sensory changes that they initially give up all hopes of ever experiencing sexual pleasure again. Instead, they may choose to focus all their energy on satisfying their partners. This type of sacrifice is certainly not necessary—with education and a little reassurance, mutual sexual pleasure is indeed still possible after a spinal cord injury.

Before an individual with SCI begins to rediscover his or her sexuality, it is important to keep in mind that sensuality and personal expression are as vital to fulfillment as the sexual act itself. The focus should be on the process, not just the outcome. Accordingly, the way someone feels about his or her sexuality and overall body image is crucial. This is—understandably—a major hurdle for most people in the first months post-injury. Their bodies have been a source of frustration; they have been damaged, then poked and prodded, tested and measured. All the hospital procedures and the need for help with personal care can result in a complete loss of privacy and a sense of being sexless. It is no wonder, then, that in the early days people coping with paralysis often admit to feeling less than desirable.

Nonetheless, before someone can truly be intimate with another human being, that person must first view him- or herself as acceptable. Just because self-care requires some assistance does not mean that personal style or extra grooming should be abandoned. And though people who use wheelchairs often (and should) choose their clothing on the basis of comfort and suitability, that doesn't mean that their wardrobe cannot also include some purely fun and sexy touches. Spending time on your appearance not only improves your self-esteem but also increases your appeal to others.

Confidence is sexy. In fact, it can be more effective than any physical ability. Moreover, reconnecting with one's sexuality after spinal cord injury helps restore a sense of personal worth and well-being. The self-esteem that comes from being involved in a mutually fulfilling sexual relationship in turn enhances a person's acceptance of disability, which then undoubtedly boosts his or her attractiveness to others. In fact, research has also confirmed that the better adjusted an individual is to his or her disability, the more active his or her sexual life will ultimately be.

The first step to reclaiming sexuality post-injury is learning how your body now responds. If possible, this type of education should begin as early as inpatient rehabilitation. The hospital, in fact, is sometimes the first place people will try self-stimulation, to see if they can still feel, have erections, or ejaculate. In other cases, a nurse might initiate a conversation about changes in sexual functioning in response to noticing a reflex erection during catheterization, for example. Most medical personnel will be able to answer any questions about sexuality. If not, clinical nurse specialists, urologists, or gynecologists are always available for more information. In addition, plenty of books, websites, and educational videos exist on the subject. Many of my patients have also found it extremely helpful to talk to other people with SCI who are comfortable discussing the issue of sexuality. These individuals have first-hand knowledge of what to expect, as well as experience with adapting to many of the same personal challenges.

Changes in Male Erectile Function

John, a twenty-six-year-old man with T12 paraplegia, had not been a very adventurous sexual partner even before the fall off a ladder that caused his injury. He basically relied on "traditional" intercourse, which he enjoyed and also seemed to satisfy his girlfriends. "I wasn't really into oral sex," he says. "I didn't have much experience, and the times I did try I didn't really get the women off. I had always been too shy to ask what someone wanted, and I was usually so horny I didn't have the patience anyway. Oral sex was OK, but most of the time I just wanted to get on to the main event."

After his injury, John worried that his days as a lover were over. "Before, I could get hard if I just thought about a girl. Now I needed to shoot some drugs into my penis to wake it up, and even then I didn't stay hard too long. The few times I tried having sex that first year, it was a disaster. The women were nice about it, but I could tell they weren't satisfied. After a while I just stopped trying."

No matter what their level of injury, most men find that they are still capable of having some sort of erection. In general, there are two types of erections: psychogenic and reflex. Psychogenic erections result from thinking about sex or hearing or seeing something that is arousing. The brain sends these arousal messages through the spinal cord to the penis, which then becomes stiff. Men with incomplete paralysis are more likely to have preserved psychogenic erections, especially if their injuries are in the higher parts of the spinal cord. They can still be aroused by emotional or mental stimulation.

Reflex erections, in contrast, occur in response to direct physical stimulation of the penis. They are involuntary and can occur without any sexual thoughts. Men with spinal cord injuries at T12 and above (that is, spinal cord damage at the level of the bottom of the rib cage and above) can usually still have these kinds of erections. Men with lower spinal cord injuries cannot. These erections depend on a reflex arc that involves the sacral cord, not the brain. Sensory information from the penis goes right to the sacral spinal cord and back again, causing this kind of an erection. Since they can happen anytime the penis is touched or rubbed, reflex erections may occur at inopportune moments, like when a man is being catheterized or bathed. Not only are they poorly sustained, but they are also a bit unpredictable; just being turned in bed can cause one to occur. With time and practice, however, most men are able to learn what kind of stimulation and positions are most likely to cause such an erection, as well as how to make it last.

Nonetheless, some men find that the ability to have an erection does not guarantee complete "sexual success." More specifically, these post-injury erections are different; they may not be dependable enough or last long enough for a positive sexual encounter. The good news is that several treatment options are available to help men enhance their erections, including a new group of medications known as phosphodiesterase-5 inhibitors (the most widely known being sildenafil, or Viagra). Other drugs in this same class are tadalafil (or Cialis) and vardenafil (or Levitra). These medications work by relaxing the smooth muscle in the penis. Once this happens, blood flows inward and an erection occurs.

Pills like Viagra need to be taken by mouth about one hour before sexual activity, and some sort of penile stimulation is then required for the erection to occur. Normal foreplay is usually adequate. Reported side effects include headaches, flushing, stomach upset, and (rarely) blue vision, but they are usually mild and occur infrequently. Because this group of drugs cannot be taken with certain others, a physician must review all medications a person is currently taking before prescribing one of them. Overall, most men with spinal cord injury who have tried drugs like Viagra and used them as recommended (that is, not more than once daily) report better-quality erections and increased sexual satisfaction.

On the other hand, these medications will not work for everyone. Some men, for instance, are unable to use them because of specific medical conditions such as high or low blood pressure or vascular disease. For others, the cost of the drug is prohibitive. While some insurance plans will pay for a certain number of pills each month, others will not cover the cost of this medication at all. As a result, penile injection therapy is the second most common treatment for erectile dysfunction, or ED. This method is popular because of the reliability and rigidity of the erections produced; it involves injecting a single medication or a combination of medications into the side of the penis with a small insulin needle. The agents used work by opening up the blood vessels in the penis and increasing blood flow.

Individuals who are trying penile injections for the first time should do so under the supervision of a physician who can properly adjust the dose and review the technique. Owing to the risk for scarring of the penis, the injections should not be performed more than twice weekly. Other possible side effects are temporary discomfort, bruising, or infection at the injection site. The most serious complication to be aware of is priapism, or a prolonged erection that doesn't go down after several hours. This condition, though rare, can be extremely painful and can damage the penile tissue; if it occurs, immediate medical attention is necessary.

Most of my patients who use this technique have told me that the biggest disadvantages are the need for hand strength and coordination, as well as good vision. This method can also take away some of the spontaneity from sexual activity. At times men who have been unable to give themselves the injections have taught their partner or attendant the technique. Yet even with some of these technical difficulties, many men still favor penile injection therapy because of the quality and predictability of the erections that occur, as well as the rapid results and relatively low cost.

Others prefer to avoid medications and injections to enhance their erections. Instead, they may opt to use a vacuum erection device (see Figure 6). With this method, the penis is placed into a vacuum cylinder and air is pumped out, drawing blood into the penis and creating an erection. A constriction ring is then placed at the base of the penis to trap the blood inside and maintain the erection. (The ring must never be left in place for more than thirty minutes at a time, because blood can clot in the penis.) Side effects with this device are uncommon but can include bruising, numbness, pinching of the scrotal tissue, and a sensation that the penis is cold. In addition, men who have some preserved genital sensation may find the apparatus uncomfortable. Although this treatment requires adequate hand function on the part of the user, battery-operated pumps are also available.

Some couples complain that the vacuum erection device does

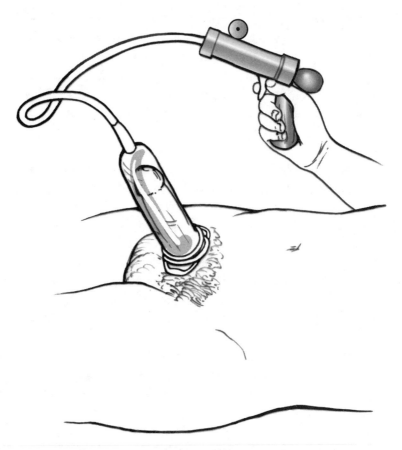

FIGURE 6.   A vacuum erection device, which uses a vacuum to draw
blood into the penis, creating an erection. This is one of several
methods to manage erectile dysfunction after spinal cord injury.

not allow for spontaneity during sex. Yet because of its general safety and low cost, many men continue to choose this
method. Moreover, this device has also been shown to give the
best-quality erections, that is, erections that are sufficiently rigid
to allow successful intercourse. The apparatus can also be used
more than once in a twenty-four-hour period and can even serve
as a backup method when other options fail.

Although they have been used less frequently since the 1980s owing to the development of less invasive and cheaper options, surgical penile implants may be considered when simpler treatments don't work. This procedure involves surgically inserting a prosthesis under the skin and into the erectile tissues to cause an erection. There are several types of systems available, but the ones that work the best for men without sensation are self-containable inflatable implants. A small pump is placed in the scrotum; when activated, it fills the penis with fluid (usually saline) and creates an erection. After sex, the implant is deflated, the fluid returns to the pump, and the penis becomes soft again.

With a variation on this option, the semirigid implant, the penis remains *partially* erect at all times. An advantage of this option over the rigid model is that the penis can be bent into different positions to make it less conspicuous when clothed. Both implant options can also be very useful for helping to keep condom catheters in place. These catheters are shaped like a condom, go over the penis, and are attached to tubing and a collecting bag. This device is useful when a person can still urinate but has no voluntary control over stopping and starting the process.

Drawbacks to penile implants include a small risk of infection and mechanical problems, as well as a slightly higher rate of erosion, whereby the prosthesis breaks through the skin. In addition, this method is generally considered permanent. Although the implant can be removed (and must be in case of infection), the device may damage penile tissue and thereby reduce erectile ability *even more* than before the implant was put in. Implants are also the most expensive option available for men, and some health insurance plans will not cover the costs. Subsequently, the various other methods available to improve erections should generally be considered before implant surgery.

As with all the other treatments, an implant will not enhance a man's sexual desire or his ability to ejaculate. Nonetheless, when they are the appropriate choice, penile implants can adequately treat erectile problems. Despite all the possible challenges associated with this method, many of my patients have reported improvements in their sex life with this surgery and seem very content with it:

"I can have sex anytime and anywhere I want, without having to bring along a pill, a syringe, or cylinder," says Larry, a single man with T9 paraplegia who has had implant surgery. "I'm able to please my partners much more, and I feel better and more confident about myself. Sure, you have to get used to it—but it was worth it for me."

Changes in Female Sexual Response

"I was sure I would never be sexually satisfied again," Robin recalls of the first months after she sustained C5-C6 tetraplegia in a car accident. "How could sex be good when I couldn't feel anything in my pubic area?"

Although sexual changes for women after spinal cord injury may not be as physically obvious as those of men, they still require adequate education and adjustment. In fact, only recently has female sexuality after SCI gained the attention of the medical community. In the past, much of our knowledge was based only on anecdotal information rather than on scientific studies. The facts were also mostly centered on menstruation and pregnancy, as little had been known about female sexual response or pleasure after paralysis.

For women who want to start or expand a family after SCI, the news is good. In contrast to injured men and their decreased fertility, women with spinal cord injuries at *any* level can still get pregnant. Some women do not get a period for the first six months after paralysis, but this is more attributable to psychological stress than to any physical changes. Consequently, any sexually active paralyzed woman who does *not* wish to become pregnant should use some form of birth control. In addition, for both men and women the risk of contracting sexually transmitted diseases is the same after injury as it was before. (This topic is covered in more detail later in the chapter.)

All women with SCI can continue to have sex regardless of the level of their injury. Although lubrication, genital sensation, and mobility may be different after SCI, none of these changes should prevent a woman from being sexually active if she so chooses. As noted, self-confidence and a willingness to experiment with sexual expression are important aspects of adapting to sexuality post-injury. Even so, some women and their partners have benefited from counseling to help them cope with the psychological aspects of these changes.

One such change involves vaginal lubrication. Just like erections, lubrication can result from thinking about sex (psychogenic) or by stimulation of the genital area (reflexogenic). Whether it will happen, and to what extent, depends upon the severity and location of the injury. If the damage is incomplete and below T12, psychogenic lubrication can occur. If the injury is higher, above T9, reflex stimulation can cause lubrication, even when the paralysis is complete.

Of course, other factors can also affect a woman's lubrication, including her mood, time in the monthly cycle, and menopause. Nonetheless, an artificial water-soluble lubricant like K-Y jelly can be helpful for lubrication difficulties. This topical gel reduces uncomfortable friction, eases intercourse, and thereby deceases the risk of infection or injury. Decreased genital sensation, limited mobility, and spasticity are other changes after spinal cord injury that may affect both female and male sexuality. (These concerns will be discussed in more detail later.)

Orgasm and Pleasure

Although few men are able to ejaculate post-injury, it is important to remember that ejaculation is not equivalent to an orgasm. In fact, about 50 percent of men and women with SCI *do* report having orgasms, independent of the level or completeness of neurological damage. Some patients have told me that for them sex is even better than before, possibly because sexual satisfaction now truly depends on both physical and psychological components. Furthermore, we know that sexual knowledge, self-confidence, a patient and inventive sex partner, and time since injury all work to enhance a person's potential for sexual pleasure and orgasm.

Despite disruptions in the nerve pathways that control the sexual organs, some men and women with SCI are still able to reach orgasm during sexual activity. Frequently, though, it takes some time for orgasms to return after injury. Yet when they do, many paralyzed people of both sexes are able to experience sensations during sexual activity that they say are "just like" the orgasms known to able-bodied individuals. Some have described sexual stimulation as causing increased muscle spasms, tingling in their legs, a rapid heart rate, and heavy breathing. Others relate no distinct physical signs but report a sense of intense pleasure, followed by a feeling of release and then relaxation. Still others relate experiencing all of the above.

As with the able-bodied community, descriptions of orgasms, as well as the mental and physical stimulation required to achieve them, vary widely from person to person. Some have explained that their bodies react to orgasms the same way they did before paralysis, but without the surface sensations. They describe the pleasurable feelings as seeming to be more internal now. One study showed that women are able to have orgasms from genital stimulation, even though they no longer have feeling in their genital area. This kind of pleasure, the research found, could also be achieved from stimulating erogenous zones. Perhaps just imagining the sensations that one can no longer feel enables some to reach orgasm. Many patients have told me that they are able to experience orgasmic sensations from stimulation to areas above their level of injury. Interestingly, many paralyzed women have also found that they now need longer periods of stimulation to achieve orgasm—an important point for their lovers to keep in mind.

Perhaps, some speculate, orgasm post-injury becomes more of a multi-sensory, whole-body experience than before. Sexual climax may now be a product of physical sensations, emotional responses, fantasies, memories of past orgasms, and—when with a partner—the excitement of connecting with another person. Regardless of what it takes to reach orgasm, the pleasure and satisfaction usually increase as people learn to relax and become more comfortable with their bodies and each other. The importance of the psychological aspects of sexual excitement should never be underestimated. In fact, they may come to be even more important than the physical aspects for those with spinal cord injuries.

Lovemaking may require some redefinition after paralysis; the key is to focus on what feels good. Many couples experiment to discover what kinds of stimulation are most pleasurable. Each partner should try to be open-minded and share his or her specific sexual desires. In an atmosphere of trust, couples are more likely to discuss their insecurities and fears, as well as the specific kinds of sensations, including sights, sounds, tastes, and touches, that they find especially pleasing.

Honest and open communication is critical to this exploration, as is some creativity, flexibility, and even playfulness to discover what works best and is most satisfying. My patients have repeatedly emphasized to me that, regardless of their physical limitations, they have still found and continue to find many ways of giving and receiving pleasure. Remember that no "rules" exist for sexual expression; the only requirement is that whatever the couple does together should be mutually acceptable and feel right to both partners.

Still, some people will undoubtedly need to change their mindset. For example, some men define their masculinity by how hard their erection is or how long it lasts, or even by the number of times they can have intercourse in one night. This kind of attitude will probably be self-defeating after paralysis. It would be far more productive for a person to concentrate on his remaining abilities rather than dwell on what has been lost.

What's right is what works *now*. Giving and receiving sensual massage, passionate kissing, cuddling, and caressing can be extremely gratifying, especially when both partners are naked and enjoying the closeness of being together. Paying careful attention to as many senses as possible can also enhance the sexual experience. Sexy clothes and soft lighting may be a turn-on for some people, while for others romantic music best sets an erotic mood. The smell of incense or fragrant candles may also make a scene more intimate.

For many people, imagination and fantasy become more important during sexual activity after SCI. Talking to each other about sensations they are experiencing may help to intensify them for a couple, and guiding a partner's hand can increase the pleasure of touch. Taking in the sights and sounds of a partner during lovemaking—facial expressions, changes in breathing—can also heighten an individual's sexual enjoyment and satisfaction. Orgasmic sex requires tuning in to the moment and putting aside skinny legs, weak muscles, or bowel and bladder problems. It means not obsessing about a partner's fulfillment or focusing on trying to reach climax alone. It is about relaxing, enjoying the sensations that *are* received, and feeling the pleasure.

*"I'd never been too much of a talker during sex, because my partner
knew exactly what it took for me to climax," says Amy. "All that
changed after I broke my neck in a car accident. Now that I had
minimal bodily sensation, we had to find new ways to make things
work. We did a lot of talking and exploring, and it turned out there
were other places on my body that could become incredibly
aroused—especially just above my nipples and around my earlobes.
By focusing all my energy on the here and now and letting her caress
and kiss me in these spots, I found I could experience a type of intense pleasure that was very similar to my old orgasms. It definitely
was more 'mental' than it ever was before, and I felt like it had
more to do with the deep connection we had as a couple than just
the act itself."*

Sexual Exploration

Discovering changes in sexuality after spinal cord injury is best
done with the right person. But the truth is, not everyone is in a
stable, loving relationship—or even wants to be. In addition,
some people may need time to feel comfortable enough with
themselves post-injury to open up and get involved with another.
With this in mind, many paralyzed people turn to masturbation to discover how they can now experience pleasure. Self-
stimulation is frequently the first step toward understanding
one's new sexuality and an excellent way to explore sexual response. It not only helps release sexual tension but can also improve the way a person feels about his or her body. This kind of
self-experimentation allows an individual to discover what works
best for him or her, information that can be communicated later
on to a partner.

People who lack hand strength can use vibrators to explore
their bodies post-injury. These devices are quite safe when operated properly, though people with injuries at the level of T6 or

above need to watch for possible increases in blood pressure that can occur with this kind of stimulation. Symptoms of this complication, called autonomic dysreflexia, include headache, dizziness or lightheadedness, and flushing of the skin. The best treatment is to stop the activity and try again at another time. (This and other complications of SCI are detailed in Chapter 11.)

Keep in mind that sexual arousal, excitement, and gratification do not have to come from the genitals alone. After spinal cord injury, stimulating many different parts of the body, even areas without sensation, can be intensely pleasurable and satisfying. While for some people only the areas with preserved sensation become supersensitive, many others find an especially responsive area right above the point where their loss of sensation begins. Some have found that, when these new erogenous zones are stimulated, the sensation is similar to that experienced preinjury when the clitoris or penis was touched. Caressing this "border zone" area can even result in orgasm. Perhaps this kind of "transfer of sensation" occurs as a result of people's memory of previous sexual feelings. Maybe paralyzed individuals are able to retrain their minds in such a way that pleasurable sensations from "ordinary" body areas now feel as if they are coming from the genitals. On the other hand, even those who have *never* experienced orgasm before they were paralyzed have related similar experiences of reaching sexual climax by having these zones stimulated.

Trying New Positions and Approaches

Because muscle weakness will affect a person's ability to get into and maintain certain body positions that have traditionally been used in lovemaking, some couples may find the need to experiment with different positions. For example, some people enjoy having sex seated in their wheelchairs with the armrests removed to allow more room to move. Others prefer lying side-by-side or face-to-face, positions that offer the most contact and the fewest balance difficulties. Some couples find that sitting up on a firm surface using pillows for support and with their legs wrapped around each other is quite pleasurable. Firm surfaces help to make transfers easier, and objects like pillows or rolled towels can be used for support. Adding rails to the sides of a bed can prevent rolling and also help with position changes. Keep in mind that loss of sensation can also make it difficult for the paralyzed partner to position himself correctly during sex. Moreover, some areas of the body may have increased sensitivity or be painful to touch and should therefore be avoided during lovemaking.

If increased muscle rigidity or spasms become problematic during sex, the couple may need to approach their movements more creatively. For example, certain positions could be more helpful in reducing muscle tone than others, like lying on your back with knees bent, lying on your side, or even getting down on all fours. Once again, experimentation is key. If spasms are still interfering with sex, relaxation techniques like massage can be a useful adjunct to foreplay. A warm shower, a little stretching, and even raising the temperature of the room can also help manage increased muscle tone. On the other hand, some people find that the spasms actually *aid* sexual movement and positioning, and even help to intensify the stimulation or trigger erections.

Oral sex often becomes a means of achieving sexual satisfaction after SCI, especially when hands are weak and erections are inadequate. This practice allows each partner to share the sensations of contact. Even when a person's genital sensation is decreased, just watching a partner perform this act can be intensely gratifying. Heterosexual men who still wish to pursue intercourse despite difficulty with erections can try a method called "stuffing." In this technique, the man stuffs his flaccid penis into the woman's vagina. This method usually works best with the woman on her knees atop the man, who is lying on his back. "Stuffing" is used primarily to give pleasure to the woman, though it may also increase the physical stimulation to the penis and thereby cause an erection. As a result, both partners may find the experience enjoyable.

Other couples use adaptive equipment to broaden their sexual expression when physical limitations get in the way. For example, vibrators can help intensify touch in parts of the body where sensation is decreased, or even in areas not considered to be erogenous zones, like the chest or neck. Vibrators may also be helpful for reaching areas that fingers cannot, and they can be adapted with straps if grip is limited. Additionally, some people experiment with various oils and lotions to enhance the sexual experience, as well as to help themselves relax and enjoy the sensuality of the moment.

Dealing with Loss of Spontaneity

Spontaneity is another major aspect of sexuality affected by paralysis. After a spinal cord injury, getting ready for sex takes more time and preparation than it used to. For example, a paralyzed person may need assistance with removing clothes, positioning, bowel and bladder care, and even birth control. Some people have their personal care attendants help them get into bed or into a specific position with a partner. Naturally, there are some drawbacks to this arrangement: The couple's lovemaking will have to be coordinated with someone else's schedule, and privacy is undoubtedly sacrificed. Yet this kind of service from an assistant can be just as important to a person's quality of life as help with showering or mobility. Help with intimate encounters is not part of a PCA's typical job description, so some diplomacy and patience will be necessary to work out all the details that may come with assuming this responsibility. Some aides may be unwilling to help, and others may only offer to assist with positioning. A few, however, have even been willing to help the disabled individual place his or her hand on a lover's body. Regardless of the specifics, all parties involved should agree on the arrangement and be comfortable with it.

Some people, of course, prefer to keep their personal care attendants completely out of their romantic affairs. If their partners are physically able, they may choose instead to train them to help with the preparation for sexual activity. Some couples have found ways to make these tasks a part of foreplay, a way to increase their bond and connection and, subsequently, the intimacy. Instead of regarding the removal of a catheter or the insertion of a diaphragm as a drawback, for example, they consider it another way to share and discover each other's particular needs.

Bowel and bladder accidents are one of the most commonly cited fears among people with spinal cord injury who are sexually active. To reduce the anxiety and possible embarrassment, I recommend that people openly discuss the issue with their partners ahead of time. This way, they will know what to expect and may even be more ready to help out. Like so many other potential problems, accidents can usually be avoided with precautionary measures. For example, because sex can increase pressure on the bladder and cause leakage, I always recommend that a person try to empty his or her bladder or use a catheter beforehand.

The same is true for the bowels: Staying on a regular schedule or doing a bowel program (for example, using a suppository to help empty the gastrointestinal tract) several hours before sexual activity will also minimize the chances for accidents. Likewise, avoiding eating and limiting fluid intake before sex can also help prevent incontinence. Yet even with these precautions, you should always be prepared for mishaps and have a urinal or towel nearby. It's also a good idea to keep protective coverings on the mattress or use absorbent pads. And when an accident does occur, a little humor goes a long way in helping ease the tension. The best thing to do is just quickly clean up and get back to the activity at hand.

Although several of my patients have voiced concerns that their indwelling catheters may interfere with sexual activity, this has not been the case for most couples. Some have found that openly discussing their catheter with their partner eliminates any surprises or discomfort, and also helps the partner understand how it works. Men can fold the catheter back over the penis and cover it with a condom to reduce friction. Women can tape the catheter to their abdomen or move it to the side out of the way. If the catheter does cause discomfort due to rubbing, extra lubrication can be used. Having extra tubing will allow plenty of room to move around. Some people choose to remove their catheters before sexual activity as long as their bladders are empty. Partners may even offer to do this themselves as a part of foreplay.

Prostitution and Sexual Surrogacy

Sometimes out of shyness, a feeling of desperation, or simply a desire to experience another form of sexual expression, some people with SCI have chosen to use the services of prostitutes. Although illegal, this route may be seen as a safe alternative for some people to learn about their "new" sexuality—especially if they feel insecure about their lack of experience. Because such interactions are often anonymous, individuals have the opportunity to engage in freer sexual exploration and gain confidence in their abilities. There is no risk of rejection, and neither party ever has to see the other again. There are certainly drawbacks to this arrangement, however. First and foremost is the risk of arrest, as the solicitation of prostitutes is illegal in most states. In addition, there is a greater likelihood of contracting sexually transmitted diseases with someone who has had multiple partners. Still, those interested in enjoying the pleasure of "guaranteed" sex with no emotional ties or commitment may be willing to take their chances.

A legal alternative to prostitution is sexual surrogacy. This is another means for a person with a new disability to explore and develop his or her sexual potential. If someone is having difficulties with physical or emotional intimacy, a licensed sex therapist may refer him to a surrogate. Once a referral is made, the therapist typically will continue meeting with the paralyzed client and the surrogate throughout their time together. Surrogates work to help clients feel more comfortable with their sexuality, improve their body image, and build sexuality and relationship skills. Surrogates use formal teaching as well as hands-on practice—everything from "sensuality exercises" that involve body touching to actual intercourse—to improve intimate expression and ease anxiety. They also help their clients learn to communicate effectively so they can enter an intimate relationship with confidence.

Unlike prostitutes, surrogates focus on education. They are professionally trained and always work in conjunction with a licensed supervising therapist. Many belong to a formal organization called the International Professional Surrogate Association (or IPSA). Additionally, unlike many encounters with prostitutes, sexual surrogacy is rarely a one-time affair: the relationship can last anywhere from a few months to several years. Moreover, all three parties (the client, the surrogate, and the therapist) must agree on how and when to end the arrangement. Above all, surrogate partner therapy is *not* a contract for sex; rather, it is a therapeutic association in which the primary focus is on relationships and intimacy. As such, it also encompasses sexuality and sexual expression.

Just fourteen when a gymnastics accident resulted in a C7-C8 frac-ture, Alan was still a virgin five years later. "I had made out with girls a few times after my injury but because I was very self-conscious about my skinny legs and paunchy stomach, I never wanted to get naked with someone else," he says. "Besides, with my unreliable erections, I never knew what was going to be going on down there."

When an old buddy from rehab told Alan about how much a sex-ual surrogate had helped him, he decided to give it a try. "I called the same sex therapist he had used, and she introduced me to Jenn," recalls Alan. "She was so cool, she put me at ease right away. We spent the first two times we got together just talking about my past experiences with girls—and my fears. Then we moved on to ac-tual touching. Jenn helped me find erogenous zones throughout my body, and by the time we actually had sex, I was starting to realize that the amount of sensation or strength I still had didn't really matter. What was important was how I was feeling about myself and my ability to be intimate with somebody else."

The Responsibilities of Being Sexual

As if there wasn't already enough to worry about, all individuals with spinal cord injuries at T6 and above need to be aware that sex and stimulation can cause autonomic dysreflexia. This con-dition (discussed in depth in Chapter 11) usually results from a full bladder or bowel, but can also be a response to sexual activ-ity. Because of the high blood pressure that may result, auto-nomic dysreflexia must be regarded as a medical emergency. The symptoms are usually headache or lightheadedness, anxi-ety, and palpitations, and may also include flushing of the skin above the level of a person's injury. If any of these occur, the paralyzed person should stop sexual activity and sit up. Once the episode resolves, physical intimacy can be resumed. If this type of problem continues to occur, however, the person should consult his or her physician for a medical evaluation. The doctor may need to prescribe drugs to prevent the increase in blood pressure.

Remember, too, that sexual activity always involves some responsibility. If a woman with SCI does not wish to become pregnant, she should use some form of birth control, since female fertility is not affected by paralysis. Finding the best method of contraception post-injury can be challenging since no method is perfect and each one has its advantages and disadvantages. Many women prefer oral contraception, or the Pill, because it is easy to use and very effective. Yet many physicians are hesitant to prescribe this medication for someone who is paralyzed, since the Pill is known to increase a woman's chance of developing blood clots. Despite this increased risk, some women still choose to use the newer low-dosage pills and "play the odds" by closely watching for any signs or symptoms of blood clots.

Many physicians also recommend that paralyzed women avoid using intrauterine devices (IUDs). The concern is that because women with SCI have decreased sensation, they may be unable to detect some of the serious complications that have been linked to this method of birth control, like infections or perforation of the uterine wall. Limited hand function can also interfere with the ability to periodically check the IUD's placement. Still, many women continue to use IUDs because of their comparatively minimal side effects, and the fact that they do not interfere with sexual spontaneity.

Barrier methods are another popular form of post-injury birth control. They include all devices that physically prevent the sperm from reaching the uterus such as the diaphragm, sponge, and condom. These are all reliable, but they have two drawbacks for people with SCI: the loss of spontaneity during sex, owing to the need for placement; and the difficulty of using them when you have decreased hand dexterity, sensation, or mobility. To circumvent this problem, devices called "inserters" are available to help with placement; alternatively, a partner can be trained in the technique. In terms of ease, condoms are certainly the best choice for birth control, and they also have the added benefit of reducing the spread of sexually transmitted diseases. Overall, no matter which birth control method a person chooses, he or she must consider all the risks and benefits.

Finally, it is important to remember that the risk of contracting and spreading sexually transmitted diseases is the same before and after injury. Specific diseases include gonorrhea, syphilis, herpes, and AIDS. These infections can cause serious medical problems, among them infertility and pelvic inflammatory disease. Preventing these infections requires understanding how they are contracted, as well as using safe sex practices with every encounter. Undoubtedly, the safest and most effective way to prevent these diseases is to use a condom correctly and with a spermicidal gel. If you're having sex with someone who has had previous partners, a condom should always be worn, even if you're also using another form of birth control. Unprotected oral sex also poses a serious risk for contracting these infections. The best prevention is an unlubricated condom, a dental dam, or even a piece of plastic wrap as a barrier between the mouth and the vagina. Overall, in order to prevent these diseases from spreading, any individual who is sexually involved, whether paralyzed or not, needs to be properly informed, receive the appropriate testing, and act safely.

Couples and Relationship Issues: Making It Work

When Meredith was in the rehab hospital recovering from the fall that left her with paraplegia, she came across some of the statistics about relationships and spinal cord injury. "They were not very supportive of marriages continuing after injury," she recalls. "The divorce rate was very high, so I took it to heart that my husband was going to leave me. I got so depressed about it that I basically said to him, 'If you're going to leave, let's get it over with right now while I'm in rehab. I don't want you staying in this marriage because you feel trapped in it. Sure, we took an oath for better or worse, in sickness or in health, but neither of us predicted this.' When he said he was incredibly insulted that I had even suggested that, it was a big relief."

Although statistics show that the majority of people who suffer a spinal cord injury are young and single at the time, those with committed life partners can face great challenges in their relationships. Just like the individual who experiences the paralysis, his or her partner is similarly affected by the changes—and losses—that come with disability. Both members of the couple will need to make major adjustments now that SCI has become part of their life together.

By contrast, when a person "marries into" disability by falling in love with someone who has an existing spinal cord injury, very different issues exist. The same sudden need for life changes does not occur because the paralysis has been a part of the partner's makeup from the start of the relationship. Couples in this situation make the deliberate choice to create a lifestyle that works for them; they have the added advantage of time to adapt to each other's differences. But when spinal cord injury is unexpected, a sudden alteration in the equilibrium of the family system results, which can either strengthen the clan's bond or cause major havoc. Although some partners are able to make it work, others are not. Regardless of their ultimate success, many couples have shown that the survival of a relationship really has more to do with the foundation two people form together and how they cope with crisis than with the injury itself.

How Couples React to Injury

In my experience getting to know couples in the hospital, a partner's reactions often parallel those of the person who is paralyzed. Although the immediate loss is undoubtedly more intense for the injured person, his or her non-disabled partner may experience many of the same emotions, concerns, and challenges. In the beginning, the future often seems uncertain for both members of the couple.

Fear and Helplessness

Many able-bodied partners report that their first reaction to the shock of new paralysis is fear; they worry that their loved one will not survive. Once the threat of death is no longer imminent, anxiety usually sets in. Many questions arise: How will our lives be changed? How much care will my partner need? Who will provide the help? How will the medical expenses be paid? Will we have to move?

Even before any of these questions can be answered, the family must learn to deal with the "new world" of the hospital, including its seemingly esoteric rules and regulations, confusing medical terminology, and numerous staff members. The separation of partners during hospitalization also adds to their stress, as does the need for the able-bodied individual to manage any family affairs single-handedly. All the usual routines have now changed, and partners often admit to feeling quite lonely upon returning to an empty home night after night until their loved one is discharged.

Some patients' significant others have complained of feeling excluded or poorly informed about what is going on during the hospitalization. This is probably because most healthcare professionals tend to focus their energy on the serious medical needs of the newly injured. Partners often voice their concerns about whether their loved one is receiving the best, or even the right, treatment. Life becomes filled with uncertainty, both about what the paralyzed individual is going through and about what lies ahead.

In addition to frustration, many significant others admit to feeling powerless because they are unable to "make it all better." Especially in the beginning, the injured person's daily routines are controlled by doctors, nurses, and therapists, sometimes with little input from the family. Although partners are encouraged to attend various therapy and educational sessions, some may find it troubling to watch their loved one trying to learn new ways to move from bed to chair or to feed themselves with adaptive equipment.

When talking to partners of the newly paralyzed, I usually recommend that they try to learn all they can about their loved one's specific injuries, which will ultimately help them gain a greater sense of understanding and control over the situation. Knowledge and communication can be important allies for managing feelings of helplessness, as can regular communication with the interdisciplinary team.

Grief

Grief is another common response among significant others of the newly disabled. They may experience sadness, not only for the losses that their loved ones have incurred, but also for the sudden transformation within their *own* lives. The entire family is affected by the decreased independence and spontaneity caused by paralysis. Significant financial changes may occur; responsibilities may shift (including jobs inside and outside the home); and even the life goals and plans of the couple may change.

While non-disabled partners are struggling to be strong for their loved ones, they are also grieving the parts of their own lives that were once taken for granted and now are gone. People usually experience this emotional vulnerability as one of two extremes: either they end up avoiding their feelings and spending less time at the hospital; or they become over-involved, helping their partners more than they should (see below). Despite their good intentions, partners may actually be doing more harm than good for their loved ones during rehabilitation.

Significant others frequently report feeling overwhelmed by their emotions. Just like the individuals who experience the paralysis, partners can benefit from the reassurance that responses like grief and despair are normal. They should be encouraged to try to experience, as well as work through, these emotions, no matter how painful, Moreover, professionals like the hospital social worker, psychologist, or chaplain can be very helpful for family members during this challenging time shortly after injury.

Guilt

Even when they have had no role in causing the paralysis, partners of people with SCI often admit to feeling guilty. While their loved ones are faced with weeks to months of hospitalization, as well as the likelihood of having to use a wheelchair from that point on, they remain able to walk around and be independent. Trying to balance the everyday responsibilities of work, maintaining a household, and taking care of children, while also finding time to be at the hospital for support and encouragement, can be an additional source of anxiety or even resentment for partners. And even though it is impossible to be two places at once, of course, they may still beat themselves up about it.

When guilt becomes overwhelming, some partners may try to be with the disabled person as much as possible. In doing so, however, they risk neglecting some or all domestic tasks, leaving bills unpaid and the house unclean. Ironically, such gestures may ultimately cause even *greater* strain on the relationship as the couple's life outside the hospital becomes increasingly disorganized.

For some partners, the result of all this guilt can be a tendency to overprotect their loved ones and do more for them than is necessary—or helpful. For example, some well-meaning family members may still feel compelled to feed their paralyzed partners, even when they have already mastered eating independently with the use of adaptive equipment. These efforts to compensate for the losses that their significant others have experienced actually *reduce* the independence of their companions. Other able-bodied people completely repress their guilt and act as if nothing has changed to protect their partners from additional worry. This approach can backfire as well, resulting in misdirected anger when deep-seated tensions eventually rise to the surface. Partners who have effectively managed their emotions have told me that they attribute their success to finding a proper balance between the roles of caregiver and significant other, then sticking with this middle road.

Frustration and Resentment

Once admitted to a rehabilitation facility, patients are faced with the prospect of an extensive recovery period—ranging from one to many months—as well as the possibility of permanent disability. The situation never seems fair, and able-bodied partners often find themselves angry and frustrated. Sometimes the anger is about the cause of the injury, especially if it resulted from an accident or a violent crime; other times family members are resentful that it happened to their loved one and not somebody else.

Occasionally, the frustration becomes too intense to hold inside any longer, and it comes out as misdirected rage. A husband, for example, may lash out at the hospital staff or doctors who are unable to make his wife better. A wife, in turn, may direct her rage at God or fate. Sometimes, if the able-bodied individual (subconsciously or consciously) feels angry with his or her partner for becoming paralyzed and indirectly causing the family upheaval, the newly paralyzed person may receive the brunt of the hostility. The able-bodied partner may even come to resent all the attention and sympathy the disabled person is given while he or she is left alone to pick up the pieces. Unfortunately, these types of reactions and the responses they elicit usually lead to further guilt and additional anger on the part of the non-injured person. The key—and the challenge—for loved ones is to find ways to direct this potentially negative energy into actions that can be both positive and productive.

Denial

For many people, the mere thought that their partner's paralysis is permanent is more than they can handle. As a result, they use denial to help them manage. They may tell themselves that the disability is only temporary or that things will soon be back to normal. Although this coping mechanism may be one way to keep from becoming overwhelmed in the short term, denial can become problematic if reality is avoided for too long.

For example, those who remain in denial may resist learning how to care for their disabled partners. They may repeatedly miss the educational sessions arranged by rehabilitation staff, or become angry at members of the treatment team who attempt to teach them about the "nuts and bolts" of paralysis. Some will even disregard the advice of therapists who recommend ways to improve the accessibility of their homes before discharge. While this kind of behavior may provide temporary protection from the emotional distress of a significant other's spinal cord injury, it may ultimately hamper rehabilitation efforts and result in bigger problems after discharge. Several partners of SCI patients have explained to me that they were not fully able to take the first steps toward adapting to paralysis until after they acknowledged their "altered reality." Only then could they start to acquire the information and skills necessary to help their loved one and adequately prepare for the life ahead.

Depression

Frequently, the cumulative result of all the emotions mentioned above—grief, anger, frustration, and guilt—is some degree of sadness. Overwhelmed by worries that a big part of their former lives is now over, partners of the newly injured may find themselves longing for the personal time and space they had before SCI. Some may start smoking and drinking more, eating and sleeping less. Others may become unable to find pleasure in *anything*, to the point where they might have difficulty getting out of bed in the morning. This sense of hopelessness can be quite debilitating, affecting their health as well as the overall well-being of their disabled partners.

Like the newly paralyzed individual who experiences clinical depression (see Chapter 3), his or her partner may also benefit from the support of a mental health professional when day-to-day living becomes difficult. Sometimes meeting one-on-one with a good counselor is all it takes to help a person develop new coping strategies for managing the situation and its accompanying stress. Many loved ones may also benefit from support groups in which they can share their experiences and learn from others who are in similar situations. Such gatherings not only allow for the open exchange of insights and ideas but also serve as a social outlet during a time when feelings of isolation are common. Those who have a biological component to their depression may additionally benefit from an antidepressant medication prescribed by a physician, though the best treatment in such cases is usually a combination of counseling *and* medication.

Many partners of the newly injured may hesitate to admit their depressed state because they feel they must support and protect their disabled loved ones. They believe that they should keep their own fears inside, lest they upset or overwhelm their companions, who already have enough on their plates. Though well intentioned, this approach can again be more detrimental than beneficial. Attempts to contain one's emotions are frequently unsuccessful, especially when a couple has been together for a long time. Furthermore, when a partner does *not* share his deep-seated feelings or the day-to-day concerns such as bills or a child's failing grades at school, the disabled partner may feel that her emotional strength has been underestimated and her role in the family devalued. At the same time, such behavior may also imply to the disabled person that she is too weak physically or emotionally to handle these matters. In reality, she may be experiencing some of the same fears as her able-bodied partner and actually be waiting for the right opportunity to discuss them with him.

Many couples have found that the most effective approach to this stalemate is open communication. Sharing their feelings gives couples an opportunity to validate each other's concerns and, at the same time, strengthen their bonds. Moreover, when they share life's everyday stresses together, partners can deepen their relationship while helping their loved ones feel connected to life outside the hospital.

Going Home

Studies have shown that individuals in committed relationships are more likely than single people to live independently after spinal cord injury. But as we have seen, this return home is usually a challenge. Paralysis does not just "happen" to one person alone; both members of a couple experience the associated changes. In this time of managed care, with shorter hospital and rehab stays than ever before, partners have less time to make the necessary physical modifications to their homes as well as the emotional adjustment to their loved one's new disabilities. How a couple reacts to these challenges depends on many factors, including individual coping styles; the understanding each person has of the injury (and the often intense feelings about the incident or disease that caused it); the number of years the partners have been together; how well they communicate; and their level of commitment and intimacy.

Some couples have told me that spinal cord injury and its effects have actually *strengthened* their bond, enabling each partner to discover and appreciate more about themselves and their significant other. This major event has also given many couples an opportunity to reexamine their values and "not sweat the small stuff." In many cases, for instance, SCI will cause people to focus more on family than ever before.

Even so, feelings of guilt, grief, anger, and resentment may resurface when the injured partner returns home. For example, accessibility issues that force a couple to pack up and move can be a significant source of stress. The challenge for the couple now is to develop coping strategies to manage the mounting uncertainty, to achieve some semblance of normalcy amid all the change, and to maintain a healthy, balanced, and fulfilling relationship.

Role Changes

No matter the circumstances, the "rules" of a relationship will usually need some reorganization when one partner experiences a spinal cord injury. Roles may change or be reversed, with the non-disabled person frequently taking on many additional responsibilities. New routines like intermittent catheterization, bowel programs, and range-of-motion exercises will have to be worked into the household's daily schedule. The non-injured partner may now have difficulty finding the additional time in an already busy day to do what used to be simple and quick—like taking a shower and getting dressed.

When the Primary Breadwinner Is Injured

For the partner who has always earned most of the family's income, a spinal cord injury that results in a temporary or permanent inability to work can be emotionally devastating. Even if his or her partner also has a job, this loss of employment can lead to anxiety and reduced self-esteem for the person with SCI. This is especially true for those who regard their jobs as a source of personal pride or status in the community. On the other hand, some individuals who are no longer able to work use these newly found free hours to help around the house and spend more time with their children and spouses. In some cases, couples have even reported *heightened* marital satisfaction after injury as a result of their increased time together.

Other injured people, however, may be unable to pitch in at

home, either because of their physical limitations or simply because they view domestic duties as "someone else's job." In
these cases, the additional time together can actually be detrimental, especially if the partner with SCI demands increasingly
more attention from his or her companion.

At the same time that a newly injured individual is suffering
from losing his or her role as breadwinner, that person's partner
could be struggling with "role overload." To maintain the financial stability of the household, for instance, a stay-at-home parent may now need to add a part- or full-time job to a list of responsibilities that already includes maintaining the home and
caring for the children. In addition, he or she may also need to
take on chores that were previously handled by the paralyzed
partner, such as yard work, snow shoveling, and car maintenance. In some cases, the non-injured companion may stop
working outside the home to concentrate on running the household and caring for his or her newly injured loved one.

Caregiver Burnout

For many partners, the addition of more work to their already
full schedule or the need to leave jobs behind leads to physical
strain and emotional stress. Able-bodied partners may try to do
too much, either out of love, guilt, or because they feel responsible for their loved one's well-being. They not only take on all the
chores of the household but also assume primary responsibility
for helping their paralyzed companion with transfers, bathing
and dressing, and even "bumping" (helping someone seated
in a wheelchair up or down stairs). For many individuals, this
amount of responsibility coupled with physical work is overwhelming.

Unfortunately, the end result is often total exhaustion and
emotional burnout. Partners may become depressed and emo-

tionally distant or resentful of the loss of control and personal time. In addition, sometimes newly disabled partners will subconsciously push their loved ones away emotionally, out of fear or guilt over their sudden dependence. Misperceiving this reaction as anger, the non-injured companions may also withdraw, believing that they have failed in the relationship. In the end, this labor of love often winds up harming not only the couple's bond but also the caregiver's health.

Many people have found that the first step toward solving this dilemma is recognizing that it exists and acknowledging the need for some sort of remedy. Since devoted partners often maintain high expectations for themselves, it may be difficult for them to admit their limitations. Many appear to view this type of role overload as an obligatory part of being in a committed relationship with a disabled partner. As a result, they overextend themselves both physically and emotionally and ultimately neglect their own needs.

More often than not, after their disabled partners come home from rehab, these caregivers will need help themselves. They should be reassured that taking time off doesn't imply that they are any less caring or devoted; rather, it means that they are able to make a realistic assessment of what they can and cannot do. Accordingly, they may also need validation that hiring outside help is more a sign of inner strength and insight than an indication of failure. More specifically, this type of action will help them maintain *their own* overall health and well-being, and subsequently ensure that they will be available to provide any assistance that their paralyzed companions may need.

The most obvious solution for caregiver burnout is either to have someone assist with the personal care of a paralyzed partner or to "outsource" some or all of the household chores. I usually recommend to patients and families that this is the time to take friends and relatives up on their offers to "help in any way we can." Any support with errands, babysitting, yard work, or even bill paying can help lighten the load. If this type of assistance is not available and finances permit, hiring outside help can be an equally effective means to give exhausted partners peace of mind and allow them to renew their energy.

With all that has to be done in a household in which one member of a couple becomes paralyzed, it is not surprising that the emotional needs of the caregiving companion can get overlooked. Because of minimal free time, social isolation, and the stress inherent in this role, caregivers are at a higher risk for clinical depression. To help battle the blues, these companions should be empowered both to take care of themselves and to spend some time away from their loved ones. I have often encouraged exhausted partners to schedule *their own* long-neglected doctor's appointments, to continue *their own* exercise regimens, and to resume *their own* hobbies. We should never underestimate the restorative powers of a long bike ride, an hour or two with a good book, or an afternoon in the garden. Furthermore, by taking steps to enjoy themselves and gain back a degree of control over their lives, they will likely be better—and happier—caregivers as well.

Another important strategy to ease the burden on able-bodied caregivers is to have the paralyzed partners do whatever they can for themselves and the household. Although some caregivers always do more than necessary out of a sense of devotion, they should be reminded that encouraging their companions' independence and participation is good for *both* parties. For example, even the most severely disabled people, though unable to help with physical chores, can remain active contributors to the household by assisting with more cerebral tasks such as balancing the checkbook, seeking out new recipes, or even taking telephone messages. Sharing the domestic responsibilities helps strengthen the couple's bond and reinforce a sense of equality in the relationship.

Maintaining outside social contacts is also extremely important for the mental health of a caregiver. Entertaining friends or visiting them at *their* homes helps to lessen feelings of isolation and loneliness, and can provide a temporary break from the daily routine. Furthermore, spending time with friends gives a person the opportunity to share his or her feelings and concerns with others who may be emotionally removed from the situation. Studies have shown that this type of companionship and encouragement can reduce anxiety and depression among caregivers—even just a phone call to an old friend can help.

Often individuals living with a disabled companion have found therapy and support groups to be extremely beneficial. In many states, local chapters of the National Spinal Cord Injury Association have such groups specifically geared to caregivers and families. Attending these meetings allows people to see that their situation is not unique. They may also be able to gain from the insights of others as they share feelings, exchange ideas, and learn new coping strategies. On the other hand, if caregivers become so emotionally overwhelmed that they no longer feel capable of providing their loved ones with the assistance they need, professional help from a psychologist, social worker, or psychiatrist may be the next appropriate step.

When the Homemaker Is Injured

For partners who are responsible for most of the household duties—including childcare—a spinal cord injury can also be a devastating blow to their self-esteem. These individuals may regard themselves as the member of the couple who "keeps things together" and "brings up the kids." Their ability to cater to the physical needs of their children—or even just lift them out of bed—may now be limited by arm and/or leg weakness. Doing the housework may become increasingly challenging as well, and this inability to fulfill their familial responsibilities may result in sadness, anger, and anxiety. These newly injured individuals may also worry that the family's needs are not being met, and that they are letting down their loved ones.

Couples in this situation usually handle the redistribution of roles very differently from households in which the primary breadwinner becomes disabled. In most cases when homemakers are injured the able-bodied partners hire outside help to care for their homes, their children, and their loved ones rather than take on these extra duties themselves. Although this type of arrangement reduces the potential strain on the household, some paralyzed individuals may resent the fact that their previously revered positions in the family are being taken over by outsiders, while their loved ones return to their regular work schedules outside the home.

By contrast, some people may readily accept that additional assistance is necessary. They recognize that their companions are returning to work either because the family needs the income or because staying at home is simply not to their liking. In such cases, the paralyzed individuals may strive to preserve their roles as much as possible, either by continuing to make homemaking decisions, for example, or by assisting with the childcare as best they can.

Once again, it is not the extent of paralysis that couples find most disruptive; rather, it is the need for changes in family roles. More specifically, many people with high tetraplegia, like Cindy Purcell, have proven extremely capable of maintaining highly organized households and harmonious relationships. Even though they themselves need the help of personal care attendants, they are able to retain their role within the family and thereby remain empowered and better able to adjust to their loss of mobility with hope and determination. They can focus on other things besides themselves and their injury. By maintaining their roles and partnerships, they have preserved their self-esteem and reduced the stress experienced by both partners.

Interestingly, studies have shown that among couples in

which the primary breadwinner can no longer continue working because of SCI, those with the most severe degree of paralysis have been able to maintain the highest level of relationship satisfaction. When, for instance, individuals have no arm or leg movement at all, their able-bodied partners have more readily accepted their need to take on additional roles, despite the added stress. In contrast, for those couples in which the injured person has far less extensive physical limitations but is neither working nor contributing to the household, the risk for conflict is much greater. Despite all the challenges of spinal cord injury, couples seem to fare better when the role adjustment or reorganization is most clearly defined and accepted by both partners.

To Caregive or Not?

For Danny, the key to keeping his marriage strong amid the challenges of his paralysis is clear: a firm dividing line. "When you marry an able-bodied person, you need to keep your spouse away from the medical ins and outs of your injury as much as possible," he says. "When you mix the intimacy of marriage with stuff like bowel and bladder care, it's a recipe for failure. The able-bodied spouse becomes burned out. Too many people mix intimacy with caregiving, and the relationship blows up in their faces. When I had a bad pressure sore and needed my wife to change my bandage twice a day, I felt during those moments like I was losing my connection as a husband—and becoming a patient."

Feelings like Danny's are not uncommon in relationships where one partner is paralyzed. Besides the physical demands and emotional stress that come with being the primary caregiver for a disabled person, there is the relationship itself to consider. Some people take on this role out of a belief that it is their duty. Others do so in order to keep all caregiving within the family, the assumption being that only they can do it right. Some family members of my patients have objected to the idea of an outsider providing intimate personal care to their loved ones; others have simply not wanted to have strangers in their homes.

Additional psychological and cultural factors may also play a role in the decision to serve as a loved one's primary caregiver. Some people may feel intense pressure to "do the right thing" and fear that *not* doing so will make them a bad partner, while others may worry how the world will judge them if they hire outside assistance. "After all," spouses tell me, "we married for better or worse. I'm not going to desert him now." In traditional heterosexual marriages, women have usually been the ones who have felt compelled to stay at home and care for their disabled husbands. When the situation is reversed, the men have frequently chosen to hire outside help to tend to their disabled wives and continue in their customary breadwinning roles, without guilt and with fewer societal repercussions.

Some people who have chosen not to become their partner's personal care attendant cite worries about sexual intimacy as a major reason. They relate concerns that emptying catheters or giving suppositories for bowel programs will interfere with their ability to feel romantic and sexual toward their companions, believing that their role will become more like that of a nurse or parent than a lover. Other times, the disabled individuals are the ones who fear that they will no longer be seen as competent sexual partners if their significant others provide such intimate personal care. Undoubtedly, a couple's sexual intimacy *will* suffer if each companion wrongly assumes that the other no longer finds him or her attractive after sharing in personal grooming or toileting tasks.

Another concern for some people is the potential loss of balance in a relationship when one individual assumes a caregiver role for the other. Disabled partners worry that they may resent this type of dependence on their companions, as the arrangement can foster a sense of inequality. In cases in which the caregiver *does* take advantage of his or her control over the other's day-to-day living, the couple's balance of power becomes further skewed. Worse yet is the situation in which the disabled partner becomes overly demanding and assumes that since her caregiver is also her significant other and lover, he would never "quit." Occasionally this presumption has proven wrong, and the personal care attendant/significant other *has* left, leading to even greater uncertainty and distress for the paralyzed partner.

Finally, there is the possibility that the able-bodied partner will take the attendant role too far, turning the act of caregiving into his or her entire reason for being. In this case, disability becomes the central focus of the relationship and may lead to an unhealthy codependence as the two companions act almost as one. Although this arrangement may work for a short time, eventually one or both individuals come to realize that the situation is detrimental to the couple, limiting their growth. At this point, the partners will frequently choose to do whatever they can to make their lifestyle more healthy and reciprocal.

In general, able-bodied partners who choose to continue as caregivers must strike a balance between their roles of significant other and attendant. Although the specific details vary from couple to couple, most agree that their success in maintaining intimacy in relationships that also involve caregiving depends on keeping clear boundaries. Having a distinct delineation of expectations and duties enables a union to grow and become stronger.

Adequate self-knowledge and strong communication skills are two other key components that these couples claim are necessary for a happy partnership. It is important, for example, that the non-injured individual be able to recognize if personal care is truly something that he or she *can* take on, not just *should* do. If it is the latter, sincere and candid discussion of all possible options is the best way to prevent feelings of guilt or resentment in either partner. For couples who decide that outside help for personal-care needs is the answer for them, the "help wanted" section in most local newspapers or disability-related publications (as well as related websites for both) is an excellent place to start. Independent Living Centers can be another helpful resource, as can hospital social workers, who are often aware of agencies that offer private-pay personal attendant services.

On the other hand, I have known plenty of partners who are natural caregivers and have been able to thrive in this crucial position. In addition to avoiding the expense of hiring assistants, keeping personal care in the family has been emotionally rewarding for both members of these couples—and has actually brought them closer. Yet even when this arrangement does work successfully, the able-bodied partner should always be encouraged to take some time off and make use of any available resources that can help prevent caregiver burnout. For example, many community hospitals and social service agencies offer workshops or support groups where caregivers can learn helpful strategies and benefit from the experiences of others. Help is also available from organizations such as the National Family Caregiver Association, which was established to offer guidance to this vulnerable group. With the appropriate resources as well as adequate communication and shared decision-making, couples should be able to figure out the best arrangement for them.

End Results: Making It Work

Despite the challenges that a new spinal cord injury can bring to an established relationship, plenty of happy, committed couples stand as proof that success is possible. Most of the people in such unions regard themselves as *total* partners, in and for life; they tend to view disability as a two-person project, not just the responsibility of the paralyzed individual. They attempt to approach situations together, sharing the problem solving as well as the decision-making. At the same time, however, they try to prevent disability and its challenges from dominating their lives.

To make it work, able-bodied partners need to learn as much as they can about their companions' differences—physical and otherwise. This happens through honest, two-way communication, as well as a willingness to be open about fears and emotions. Once such knowledge is gained, comfort levels will usually increase, and able-bodied partners will find it easier to focus on their companions as "regular" people who happen to be paralyzed.

Although the happiest couples stress the importance of minimizing the effects of SCI in day-to-day living as much as possible, they also agree that some sort of adjustment to their lifestyles and relationships is necessary. By recognizing the true needs of the disabled partner, as well as the realistic ability (or *inability*) of that person's mate to help out, the couple minimizes the chance for misunderstandings.

Melissa had been married for five years when a car accident left her with C6 tetraplegia. After getting past the initial shock of the situation, her husband, Arthur, was able to become her primary means of emotional and physical support. Whether she needed a sandwich or a shower, he was there with a kind word and soft touch. In time, the couple came to look at such tasks not as a burden but rather as an opportunity to be together. "Our relationship is no longer defined by my injury," Melissa explains. "It's now simply one part of our life."

Accommodating Each Other

In relationships that work, able-bodied people can look beyond weakened limbs and wheelchairs to see the true essence of their partners. They are able to express pride in the accomplishments of their loved ones with SCI, whether the feat is getting back into the community, returning to work, helping with childcare, or simply living each day as well as possible.

Melissa, Arthur notes, is "just as great a wife and mother as she's always been. Even though it's pretty tough for her to play catch with our girls or do arts and crafts with them, she still helps out at their Brownie meetings. Although I've taken over the cooking duties, she's still the one who plans the menu each night and makes sure I don't burn anything. And, most importantly, she still has her same great love of life."

Honesty, compromise, and open communication are crucial to relationships interrupted by disability. Given the tremendous number of changes that such couples experience, the physical and emotional accommodations that are made must be acceptable to both individuals. Flexibility and patience are key. If at any point a situation arises that makes one person uncomfortable or frustrated, an insightful partner will be able to recognize it with little or no prompting and act accordingly. After all, no two people, whether able-bodied or disabled, can live together harmoniously if either of them lets fear, anger, or resentment brew.

Surviving the Rough Spots

Even the happiest couples admit that every relationship has its difficult moments. In fact, this very realization contributes to the success of these unions. True partners work as a team and accept each other's flaws and differences. Moreover, those facing the challenges of disability often utilize the same coping strategies that work for able-bodied couples. Humor and self-deprecation, for example, help many of them smooth out the rough spots. Rather than lamenting over inaccessible restaurants or bladder accidents, they are able to make a quick joke or two and thus turn a day ruined into a day enjoyed. One couple I know has found a surefire way to resolve any moment of tension between them: they simply stick their tongues out at each other.

Finding a balance between time spent together and time apart is another successful approach to maintaining a strong union. Although paralyzed individuals may understandably feel the need for more attention and togetherness post-injury, their able-bodied companions should also remember to preserve some of their own space so as not to feel suffocated. Of course, finding time to be *together* outside the home—whether for a romantic dinner and movie or just for a leisurely stroll—remains another important element in "keeping the spark alive" for all couples. Socializing with friends and family is also beneficial for maintaining a healthy relationship no matter the circumstances.

Reinventing a Sex Life

Physical connection is an important aspect of any solid union. In addition to being a way to share intimacy and passion, sexuality allows couples a unique means of personal expression, regardless of the strength of their limbs.

Couples dealing with SCI should accept from the outset that sex will be different now. Just like the paralysis itself, the resulting change in sexual function (discussed in Chapter 6) is a real loss that should be grieved through open discussion and, when necessary, tears. This process will make it easier for a couple to take the next step: working toward the formation of a renewed and mutually gratifying physical relationship.

During this period of adjustment, able-bodied lovers should be aware that their partners may be anxious about changes in their bodies and question whether they are still desirable. Even those in long-term, monogamous relationships may fear rejection in the aftermath of SCI. It is best to deal with these worries head-on; if not, such insecurities can lead to alienation and accusations of infidelity. Some newly disabled individuals have even confided to me that they avoid discussing sexual changes with their partners out of fear that they might turn them off or overwhelm them. The challenge for their able-bodied lovers is to help them see that, in reality, the opposite is true: This kind of candor and sincerity about feelings and needs should serve to *increase* their attractiveness, not lessen it.

Another hurdle for couples to get past is the fear of injury during sexual activity. Being disabled does not increase a person's risk of being hurt during sex, but this is nonetheless a common apprehension for those reestablishing intimacy. Some education and reassurance can alleviate these concerns; otherwise, the resulting anxiety may hamper even the strongest passion.

Once sexuality has become part of a couple's life again, some issues may still need to be resolved. The disabled lover, for instance, may have a difficult time asking for help with positioning during intimate moments. This can be especially true for those who were accustomed to taking the lead during sexual encounters pre-injury. And even when able-bodied partners have learned that neither lubrication nor erection is necessary for their paralyzed lovers to experience pleasure, some may still feel inadequate, believing that they are unable to "turn on" their companions. Others may feel guilty because they assume that they are the only ones receiving physical gratification. Yet this is often not the case at all—people with spinal cord injuries remain capable of sexual satisfaction, both through their own fulfillment and by pleasing their partners.

As with all other relationship issues discussed in this chapter, professional guidance is available for those couples unable to reach their own resolution surrounding intimacy. A psychologist, social worker, or other mental health professional can help address concerns by facilitating communication and providing both education and supportive counseling. Couples who are open to therapy are those most likely to "make it work" in the end, finding the greatest satisfaction, sexual or otherwise, in their lives together.

When Things Don't Work

Although some studies have shown that divorce is more common after spinal cord injury, the rates quoted vary greatly, ranging from 8 to 48 percent of couples. Although the likelihood of divorce seems to be greatest during the first few months after injury, rates do eventually decline to levels that are similar to those of the general population. In fact, the overwhelming majority of individuals remain married one year after SCI.

Still, given the many challenges that come with paralysis, as well as the efforts needed to make *any* relationship succeed, it is no surprise that some couples do not make it. Some individuals will blame the paralysis for the couple's problems, but a strained relationship is usually more about the personalities of the people involved and the honesty and openness (or lack thereof) that they contribute to the union.

In fact, many of these same unsuccessful relationships would not have survived even in the absence of spinal cord injury. If a solid foundation does not exist beforehand, disability will only further complicate a couple's problems. Unions that may be primarily based on physical attraction or sexual prowess, for instance, may not be strong enough to survive the frequent ups and downs of disability. In other cases, a breakup may have more to do with a specific individual's character than with any issue between that person and a spouse.

Some newly disabled individuals may also continue to harbor anger and resentment about their situation and subsequently not be able to adjust adequately to all the changes that come with paralysis. Such unresolved inner conflict may also impede a person's ability to share his life with someone else, no matter how strong his feelings are for his loved one. Alternatively, an able-bodied partner who constantly questions his or her ability to cope with a lover's situation or to handle the discrimination that frequently accompanies disability will also threaten the stability of a union. In any case, when problems arise and either person is unwilling to seek professional guidance, especially when the other feels it is necessary, the result may be an impasse.

Benefits of Committed Relationships

Despite the ups and downs that a couple faces in the years after spinal cord injury, many people have found that being in a committed relationship is well worth the effort. Disability has even *enhanced* the quality of many such unions. By experiencing this life-altering event and learning to handle its challenges together, two individuals may become closer than ever. (Even struggling together with insurance companies to secure payment for certain services or equipment can be a bonding experience.) Some couples have told me that dealing with disability only reaffirmed their commitment to and love for each other, not only through a greater appreciation for their partner's support and inner strengths, but also through the increased time they now have to spend together.

Moreover, studies have shown that individuals with spinal cord injury who are involved in monogamous relationships rate their own adjustment to disability as higher than those who don't have such partners. This "attached" group is also more likely to be gainfully employed and enjoy a highly active social life. In some cases involvement in a satisfying partnership enhances a person's potential for returning to work, while for others having a job helps to make them more desirable. Not surprisingly, disabled people with committed, loving partners have also reported a higher level of satisfaction with their sexual and social lives, living arrangements, and general health. Moreover, they profess to a greater sense of control over their lives.

The importance of maintaining healthy love relationships for one's quality of life cannot be overestimated, especially after a dramatic event like spinal cord injury. In addition to the benefits just mentioned, being connected with another human being often allows people to shift their focus from themselves and their disability as they begin "living life" again. Although making any committed relationship work takes time, energy, and above all love, the nurturing, mutual respect, unconditional acceptance, and pleasure that result make the efforts worthwhile. As many happy and successful couples have shown, once two people decide they genuinely want to be together, physical disability—even the most severe—can do little to break their bond.

Fertility and Pregnancy:
The Possibilities

Married for five years, Mark and Candace had great jobs and had just moved into a new house in the suburbs. Next on the agenda was starting a family, but their plans were put on hold when Mark was involved in a high-speed car accident that fractured his T9 vertebra. After being stabilized at a small community hospital, he underwent surgery on his spine. Shortly thereafter, he was told that he was paralyzed and would probably never walk again—or father children.

"We were devastated, but we got a lot of help moving forward with our lives," Candace recalls. "Mark spent the next three months in a rehab hospital learning how to manage in a wheelchair, while I worked with several contractors to make our house accessible for him. His boss and colleagues were very supportive and set up a revamped workspace for him when he was ready to go back to his accounting job a few months after his discharge. Then, once we had two steady incomes coming in, we couldn't help starting to think about having kids again."

Despite Mark's initial prognosis, the couple quietly began talking later that year with Mark's doctors and researching the most updated information available about fertility after paralysis. They were encouraged by what they learned. "Mark tried using a vibrator that his urologist recommended in order to obtain ejaculate, but that didn't work. A guy Mark knew from rehab and his wife had gotten pregnant using electroejaculation, so we got in touch with a fertility clinic to give that a try. We timed our visits with my menstrual cycle, and I was also closely monitored with ultrasounds and medication. It took three tries, and it was stressful, but it worked. We now have a beautiful, healthy son named Ethan, with plans to give him a brother or sister in a couple of years."

Being paralyzed does not usually change a person's desire to become a parent. And given that most people who experience spinal cord injuries are between the ages of eighteen and thirty, the prime years for childbearing, fertility may be a major concern. Whereas women experience little change in their ability to conceive after SCI (as discussed later), the same is not true for men. Most injured men are still able to have some sort of erection, but less than one in ten will be able to ejaculate during intercourse. Normal ejaculation requires a very well coordinated combination of neurological signals from multiple levels of the spinal cord, and this process is usually interrupted by paralysis.

Moreover, even when ejaculation *is* possible, only 10 percent of couples with an injured male partner are able to conceive. There are two major obstacles to achieving pregnancy for paralyzed men: their sperm has a decreased ability to fertilize eggs, and there is greater difficulty obtaining ejaculate in the first place. The good news, however, is that with technological advances in assisted reproductive technologies (ART), more and more men with spinal cord injuries like Mark are able to be fathers.

In the twenty-first century, women, too, should not be deterred from the idea of pregnancy and parenthood after SCI. For a mother-to-be who receives the appropriate monitoring from an obstetrician familiar with her particular situation, paralysis should have little impact on pregnancy, labor, and delivery. Although there may be some roadblocks along the way, many women have shown that, with commitment and adaptability, successful pregnancies are indeed possible (and increasingly common). Perhaps, most important, the babies of men and women with SCI are at no increased health risk, and the incidence of birth defects in these children is no higher than in the general population. Birth weights are also typically within normal ranges. As with much else that they have encountered post-injury, paralyzed men and women have shown that they are quite capable of overcoming any potential obstacles to parenthood.

Male Fertility Concerns

Given the many variables involved, a team approach is recommended when offering fertility assistance to paralyzed men and their partners. The team should include a urologist who can manage and optimize the injured man's urological function; a physiatrist to oversee his basic medical care related to spinal cord injury; and a gynecologist to evaluate and/or treat the female partner's needs as necessary. Rounding out this interdisciplinary team is the andrology lab worker who performs the special treatments required to prepare sperm for insemination and ensure that it is of the highest quality possible. In addition, many couples choose to consult a social worker who can help them manage the emotional roller coaster that often ensues during this stressful period.

As they work closely with this group of specialists, couples should make it a priority to educate themselves about the various methods available to obtain ejaculate, as well as the financial and medical issues involved. Possible treatments include intra-uterine insemination (commonly known as IUI) and in vitro fertilization (IVF). Having all their questions answered should help couples feel more prepared to decide on the treatment approach that best suits them, and how long to try it before moving on to another method, if necessary.

Methods of Obtaining Sperm

VIBRATORY STIMULATION

Most men who wish to obtain ejaculate, either for testing or for conception with a partner, start with the vibratory stimulation method. This is the simplest, least invasive, and cheapest available technique. A physician-recommended vibrator, with a specific frequency and strength, is applied to the head of the penis in order to stimulate ejaculation. (This method can be used even when the individual is unable to have an erection.) For best results, specialists recommend that men wait at least six months post-injury before trying this procedure. For men with complete paralysis at the T10 level and higher, or any incomplete injuries, ejaculation rates with this method are between 60 and 70 percent.

The first time a man uses vibratory stimulation should be in a doctor's office. This is because, for people with injuries above T6, the procedure carries a risk of autonomic dysreflexia, a potentially dangerous condition causing elevations in blood pressure that can lead to seizures, stroke, or even death if not managed properly (see Chapter 11). Medical personnel can provide the proper monitoring and, if necessary, prescribe drugs that will prevent the harmful rise in blood pressure. In addition, some paralyzed men using vibrators may experience "retrograde ejaculation," in which semen goes backward into the bladder instead of leaving the urethra. Because the acidic environment of the bladder is known to reduce sperm mobility, in such cases professional assistance is necessary to retrieve, wash, and prepare the sperm, as well as to assist with insemination of the female partner.

Once it is clear that neither autonomic dysreflexia nor retrograde ejaculation is a concern, vibratory stimulation can be safely continued at home. Vibrators that are specifically designed for home use are now available; these models are both powerful enough to trigger ejaculation and also approved by the Food and Drug Administration (FDA). Many men who have tried vibro-ejaculation at home recommend using the vibrator for a maximum of ten minutes, then taking a rest before another attempt. This approach helps to alleviate potential hazards of the procedure such as skin breakdown, bruising, or bleeding. Several of my patients have found that waiting a few days between sessions increases their chances for success.

Although the process is inherently unromantic, many patients tell me that they use scented candles or sensual music to help set the mood. Several men have related that the increased muscle tension in the abdomen, hands, and other parts of the body caused by vibratory stimulation can create a sort of sexual excitement. Some have even stated that when that tension is released, either through intense leg spasms that shake the entire body or through ejaculation, the experience sometimes feels like an orgasm.

When vibration works, the ejaculate should be collected in a cup and used to inseminate the female partner. At home, couples need only a syringe with a plastic plunger (and no needle) to transfer ejaculate into the vagina. Some women prefer to place the semen directly into a diaphragm or cervical cap to help the sperm enter the cervix. It is also recommended that the woman remain on her back with knees bent upward for twenty minutes after insemination, so gravity can help move the sperm along.

After waiting a minimum of two weeks, couples can then take a pregnancy test.

ELECTROEJACULATION

Although studies have shown that the quality of sperm is higher with the use of vibratory stimulation, this method will not work for everyone. When it doesn't, men can turn to electroejaculation. Success rates of 80–90 percent have been reported using this technique, with the best results noted in men with thoracic levels of injury rather than cervical or lumbar levels. In contrast to the vibratory method, however, electroejaculation must always be done in a doctor's office. Not only does it require specialized equipment, but the blood pressure of certain patients must be closely monitored every session owing to the increased risk of autonomic dysreflexia with this kind of stimulation. In fact, before this procedure is performed, many clinics give all men who are paralyzed at or above the T6 level a medication to lower their blood pressure as a precautionary measure.

Once blood pressure monitoring begins, a physician places a probe into the man's rectum and then uses an electrical current to stimulate the nerves that control ejaculation. Although the current is low, it is quite strong. As a result, those individuals who still have feeling in the rectal area may need some kind of anesthesia to tolerate the procedure. Electroejaculation also requires the presence of two nurses or assistants, one to monitor blood pressure and the other to "milk" the penis and collect the ejaculate. As with vibratory stimulation, the semen may go backward into the bladder. If this occurs, medical personnel will need to collect it with a catheter after the procedure in order to inseminate the woman. Possible complications of electroejaculation include burns or perforation of the rectum, but both are quite rare. Autonomic dysreflexia, a more common occurrence, is easily managed when the risk is identified.

Other Ways to Obtain Sperm

Men whose paralysis affects the nerves that control ejaculation or who have some sort of structural blockage are usually unable to ejaculate with either the electroejaculation or the vibratory stimulation methods. In these cases, physicians may use a needle to acquire sperm directly from the *vas deferens*, the structure where it is stored. The drawbacks to this procedure include a risk of scarring (due to the small incision) as well as the limited number of sperm that can usually be retrieved. Although this technique is not yet widely used, the hope is that with continued improvements, it will be more readily available.

Men for whom multiple attempts at ejaculation and/or insemination fail have yet another alternative: the use of donor sperm. Moreover, if they are able to obtain *some* of their own ejaculate, this can be mixed with the sperm of anonymous donors to increase their chances for conception. Some men may even use the sperm of a close family member, like a brother, as the donor. With this method, the donor sperm may fertilize the egg, or somehow provide the additional help that the prospective father's own sperm needs to "get the job done."

Sperm Quality

Besides having difficulty obtaining sperm, men with spinal cord injuries usually face another obstacle in the road to achieving a pregnancy: getting sperm to an egg so fertilization can take place. Although their sperm volume and numbers may be normal, the motility (the percentage of moving sperm) is usually low. More specifically, while 60 percent motility is considered normal, men with SCI usually have between 5 and 10 percent. Further complicating matters is that even when these sperm are capable of "swimming" to the egg, they tend to be fragile and lose their motility rather quickly.

Despite all the research focused on fertility after paralysis, the reason for the reduced sperm quality is not completely clear. Many possible causes for the motility problem have been considered, however, including medication effects or hormonal changes. Some researchers have postulated that sperm may be damaged because of the frequent infections of the bladder, prostate, or seminal vesicles (the structure where sperm are stored) that paralyzed individuals experience. Immobility and the higher scrotal temperatures that result from prolonged sitting have also been implicated in reduced sperm quality.

On the brighter side, researchers have found that men who use intermittent catheterization tend to have more productive sperm than those who have indwelling catheters or use other methods to manage their bladders. In addition, sperm retrieved by vibroejaculation tend to have better motility than sperm obtained by electroejaculation, possibly because more retrograde ejaculation and subsequent damage to the sperm occur with the latter technique. Repeated vibratory stimulation has also been shown to improve sperm quality; after weekly sessions over a three-to-six-month period, sperm motility improved to 20 percent in one study, giving couples yet another reason to continue trying despite a lack of early success.

Because of concern about fertility, several of my young male patients have asked about the possibility of "banking" (or freezing) their sperm shortly after injury so it can be used later. They assume that the quality of their ejaculate—and, subsequently, their chance for conception—will deteriorate with time. In reality, however, sperm banking immediately after paralysis is not recommended for several reasons: ejaculates are most easily obtained around six months after injury; the very process of freezing and thawing can harm the sperms' motility; and studies have shown that for approximately two years after injury, the quality of ejaculate does not significantly change. In many instances men who have been paralyzed for ten years or more (including some of my patients) have been able to ejaculate, produce adequate-quality sperm, and father children.

Assisted Reproductive Technologies (ART)

In traditional insemination, sperm is simply placed inside the vagina. It then finds its own way toward the fallopian tubes, where, it is hoped, it meets the egg. When motility is at less than normal levels, as it is for men with SCI, the odds for successful fertilization are greatly reduced. Recent advances in ART have enabled many couples to overcome this obstacle and become pregnant. For example, in IUI, a procedure frequently done in conjunction with electroejaculation, a medical professional uses a small catheter to place the sperm directly into the uterus at the most fertile time of the woman's menstrual cycle. This process greatly improves the chances that sperm and egg will meet and form an embryo. Although it is a relatively simple procedure, sperm quality must still be high enough for success to occur. According to studies, pregnancy rates for partners of men with spinal cord injury whose sperm have at least 33 percent motility and who use IUI are approximately 10–14 percent.

Couples seeking to increase their odds for conception may opt to pursue in vitro fertilization, previously known as the "test-tube baby" method. Success rates for this procedure, in which eggs and sperm are combined outside the body in the laboratory, have reached as high as 25 percent. If fertilization occurs, the resulting embryo is placed back into the uterus. IVF, because it is more technologically sophisticated than IUI, can also be quite costly depending on the couple's medical insurance and the state in which they live. (Several states, including Massachusetts and Illinois, require insurance carriers to cover ART services.) As with IUI, the success of IVF depends on both the man's ability to produce a sufficient quantity of viable sperm and his partner's age and fertility status.

When low sperm count *and* decreased motility account for fertility problems, couples may consider a new technique called intracytoplasmic sperm injection (ICSI). ICSI involves injecting a single sperm directly into an egg under microscopic guidance and then implanting the fertilized egg in the uterus. Pregnancy rates with this approach have paralleled those of IVF; yet unlike the other procedures, only a few sperm are needed.

Learning to Cope

Whatever option they choose in pursuit of pregnancy, couples with at least one paralyzed partner must be prepared to deal with all the waiting, multiple evaluations, endless monitoring, and possible disappointments inherent in this process. Even in the twenty-first century, with so many improvements in available fertility treatments, pregnancy rates for these families remain low. Couples should also realize that the entire experience, even when successful, can take two or more years. The costs in terms of emotional stress, time, and money can be a considerable drain on anyone. Yet armed with a full understanding of the available options, as well as realistic expectations and patience, couples may have an easier time coping through this often trying ordeal.

The good news is that about 40 percent of paralyzed men who have attempted to father children in the past three decades have been successful, and most of these dads say the trials and tribulations are well worth it. With continued advances in science and general knowledge about the effects of spinal cord injury on fertility, the hope is that we can develop techniques to boost sperm quality so that more of these men will be able to fulfill their goals of parenthood.

Pregnancy Challenges for Women

Sarah, a twenty-eight-year-old wife and the mother of a three-year-old, was paralyzed in a skiing accident. Although caring for her son, John, from a wheelchair could be challenging, advice from other disabled moms and a lot of patience and determination enabled her to get through—and even enjoy—his toddler years. Now, Sarah believed, John was ready for a sibling, and so were she and her husband.

Women like Sarah do not have to give up their dreams of pregnancy and childbirth. Although many assume that paralysis will affect their ability to conceive, female fertility after spinal cord injury is, for the most part, unchanged. Since stress of any kind (physical or emotional) has the potential to disrupt *any* woman's menstrual cycles, many find that their menses are temporarily interrupted post-injury. Yet because menstruation is controlled by hormones and not by the neurological system, neither the level of injury nor the completeness of paralysis will affect this process. Furthermore, after an average of six months, most women resume normal monthly menstrual cycles. When this happens, a woman's fertility returns to what it was pre-injury.

Knowing the Risks, Coming to Term(s)

Often the greatest initial obstacle to motherhood is finding health-care professionals experienced in the management of pregnancy as well as labor and delivery in women with SCI. Once a woman finds a competent doctor who is comfortable with the situation, she should be reassured that pregnancy is indeed possible—and that more and more paralyzed women are conceiving, carrying their babies to term, and having normal spontaneous vaginal deliveries. Although post-injury pregnancies do carry a risk for more complications, outcomes for both mothers and their infants are excellent, provided that the moms are in good general health and receive close monitoring. More specifically, miscarriages, still births, and intrauterine growth retardation are no more common in women who are paralyzed than in able-bodied women, nor is preeclampsia (pregnancy-induced high blood pressure). Subsequently, no extra monitoring is necessary for these specific conditions.

Because of the potential problems that paralyzed women may face during pregnancy, as well as the multiple medications that many take every day, it is important to have a thorough medical evaluation before conception. Moreover, because some drugs are best avoided during pregnancy, a physician should review all medications a woman is taking and make recommendations about which ones should be stopped or changed. Blood counts, skin condition, and bowel and bladder habits should also be assessed for any pre-existing problems. Counseling about proper diet and vitamin supplementation should begin as well.

Just like any woman who becomes pregnant, a mother-to-be with spinal cord injury should familiarize herself with the many changes—physical, hormonal, and emotional—that occur during this forty-week process. Almost all organ systems are affected in some way, and these alterations may be more pronounced in paralyzed women. The usual pregnancy-related decreases in blood pressure, for example, may be more challenging for women with spinal cord injury who already have difficulty with this issue. If this is the case, they must pay greater attention to their fluid intake and use compression stockings to help maintain their blood pressure. Similarly, the constipation that is characteristic of most pregnancies may be even more problematic for a woman whose bowels are affected by SCI. Here, the solution can be an increase in dietary fiber, laxatives, or fluids, or even a more frequent bowel program.

Weight-Gain Concerns

Although weight gain during pregnancy is a reality for all women, those who use wheelchairs have an even greater likelihood of adding extra pounds. Their increased girth may also worsen the indigestion and heartburn typically experienced by expectant mothers as the growing uterus presses up on the stomach and irritating digestive fluid backs up into the esophagus. Moreover, women with cervical or high thoracic injuries may find that their larger size and expanding uterus affect their ability to breathe easily, though in most cases proper positioning and adequate rest are usually enough to prevent serious problems like pneumonia. For those with chronic pain, additional pounds may increase the overall load on skeletal joints, adding to discomfort and making transfers and positioning more difficult.

Skin Breakdown

Skin breakdown is a preventable complication of spinal cord injury, and it should be equally avoidable during pregnancy. Close attention needs to be paid to a woman's blood counts, since anemia (a reduction in blood cells) is common during this period and can increase the risk for pressure sores. Women should also be aware that iron supplements, which are frequently prescribed for some types of anemia, will also usually worsen constipation. Weight gain is an additional culprit here; as the pressure on the buttocks and hips increases and dependence during transfers and ambulation grows, skin breakdown is also more likely to occur. Pregnant women therefore need to be even more diligent than usual with their pressure relief and skin monitoring.

Engaging in additional upper-body exercise to strengthen the arms is another way to counteract extra pounds and ease transfers. As always, added attention to proper nutrition and hydration is key to ensuring healthy skin and circulation. No matter what precautions they take, however, some expectant moms may still need wider wheelchairs, more cushioning, or transfer aids like sliding boards or trapezes to help ease mobility and relieve pressure. If any skin breakdown does occur, immediate medical attention is paramount to prevent an infection that can be harmful to both the mother and the developing fetus.

Bladder Issues

As the uterus grows, a pregnant woman with spinal cord injury may experience increased difficulty in fully emptying her bladder. As a result, urinary tract infections are often the most common complication during pregnancy. Some women also note increased urine leakage, which is best treated by catheterizing more often or switching to indwelling catheters, though both options tend to heighten the chance for infections.

Because many antibiotics can be dangerous for the growing fetus, preventing infection is the best approach. More specifically, pregnant women should be sure to drink enough fluids to keep the bladder "flushed out" and minimize any residual urine left in it. Some experienced moms swear by cranberry juice and vitamin C to keep the bladder bacteria-free. When bladder infection does occur, the appropriate treatment will prevent bacteria from reaching the kidney and upper tracts and possibly causing more serious complications like kidney failure or premature labor. If necessary, obstetricians can prescribe antibiotics that are safe for pregnant women to take.

Blood Clots

All women have an increased tendency to develop blood clots during pregnancy; for those with SCI, decreased mobility further adds to the risk. These clots (blockages known as deep venous thromboses) usually form in the veins of legs but can also travel to the lungs (as pulmonary embolisms), which can be life-threatening. All paralyzed individuals and their families need to be aware that any increased warmth, redness, or swelling in a leg can indicate the presence of a blood clot. If such a clot extends to the lungs, shortness of breath or chest pain can occur suddenly. And if *these* symptoms are noted, immediate medical attention is necessary. Once the appropriate testing confirms the presence of either of these complications, intravenous heparin (a blood thinner) is the treatment of choice; it is safe during pregnancy, as it does not cross the placenta.

Spasticity

Because several of the medications used to treat spasticity in paralyzed individuals can pose risks to a developing fetus, physicians will usually taper and stop these drugs during pregnancy. As a result, many women will experience increased muscle tone. The recommended management of spasticity for expectant moms is regular range-of-motion and stretching exercises, as well as proper positioning. If a woman experiences any sudden, unexplained increase in spasticity, however, careful medical attention is warranted since it may signal the onset of a urinary tract infection, constipation, a new pressure sore, or even labor.

Labor and Delivery

ONSET OF LABOR: DETECTION, POSITIONING

As long as a paralyzed woman has no other health concerns, she is just as likely to carry her baby to term as her able-bodied counterparts. Although the rate of preterm delivery may be slightly higher than that of the general population (some 5–10 percent of all live births), it is still lower than that of other high-risk groups, such as women who have had previous preterm deliveries. A bigger concern for pregnant women post-injury is that, because of their reduced sensation, the onset of labor may go unrecognized.

What paralyzed moms-to-be need to know is that while uterine contractions experienced by those with sensory loss below the T10 level will feel different from those of other individuals, most women with SCI have been able to perceive labor in *some* way. Some have reported the presence of abdominal tightness, increased bladder pressure, or backache as signals that labor is beginning. (Women who have preserved sensation and strength in their hands can be taught to detect their contractions through appropriate examination of their abdomens.) Others have experienced difficulty breathing or just noticed a sense of heightened anxiety that has sent them to the hospital for evaluation and, soon thereafter, delivery. One of my patients noted the sudden onset of an autonomic dysreflexia episode (see next section) that could not be explained by any other reason. When she arrived at the hospital, her labor had begun.

Because of concern for unattended delivery in women who are unable to reliably sense their contractions, obstetricians may advise that such individuals have weekly office evaluations after twenty-eight weeks (two months earlier than for able-bodied women) and possibly consider hospitalization after thirty-six weeks. Some physicians recommend that women with high levels of paralysis rent machines to monitor their uterine contractions at home.

Overall, since labor and delivery should be minimally affected by spinal cord injury, the usual obstetrical standards can be used to determine the course of action. For long labors, however, frequent position changes may be needed to avoid skin breakdown. The average length of labor and the rate of cesarean sections have been found to be no different in paralyzed women than in their able-bodied counterparts, except when the presence of a pelvic deformity or breech baby would make vaginal delivery exceptionally difficult or dangerous.

DYSREFLEXIA

For women with injuries above T6, autonomic dysreflexia is the major concern during labor and delivery. Because of this possible complication, obstetricians prefer to avoid inducing labor in such individuals. Even though paralyzed women may be unable to feel their uterine contractions in the usual sense, the central nervous system stimulation from this muscular activity, along with the passage of a baby through the widening birth canal, can lead to this potentially life-threatening condition in which blood pressure rapidly rises and heart rhythms can become irregular. As mentioned previously, if dysreflexia goes untreated, fetal distress, seizures, strokes, or even death of the mother can occur. As a result, all women who are susceptible will have their blood pressure closely monitored during labor and delivery.

If dysreflexia *does* occur, all easily treatable causes, such as bowel or bladder distension, should first be eliminated. Sometimes simply lowering the rate of intravenous fluids being given or emptying the bladder may be all that is necessary. If blood pressure still continues to rise, however, short-acting medications to lower it can be given. Overall, the best way (as always) to manage dysreflexia is to "remove the noxious stimulus" or—in this case—deliver the baby. Epidural anesthesia or spinal blocks are performed to decrease any further stimulation to the central nervous system, thereby removing the source of dysreflexia. In fact, many physicians will choose to perform these procedures early in labor for *all* paralyzed women at risk for dysreflexia as preventative measures.

DELIVERY

Obstetricians need to resort to an operative (or cesarean section) delivery when blood pressure remains dangerously elevated despite anesthesia and medications. Otherwise, since hormones and not the neurological system control uterine contractions, paralyzed women—even those with quadriplegia—should be able to deliver vaginally. Only rarely are forceps or vacuum extraction needed to help push the baby out of the birth canal. Likewise, episiotomies are seldom necessary, since the looseness of paralyzed muscles tends to lessen the risk for tears. When episiotomies *are* done, women must practice standard skin care with warm sitz baths and frequent cleansing of the area to optimize healing and prevent infection.

SCI and Pregnancy: Two Couples' Stories

Meredith and Dylan

Meredith and Dylan had been married for two years and were thinking about starting a family when a freak fall into shallow water left Meredith with L1 incomplete paraplegia. Although doctors informed her that the accident would have no affect on her ability to have children, she quickly discovered during her two-plus months in a rehabilitation hospital that there was very little information available to women with spinal cord injury who were interested in motherhood. "We spent hours talking about semen production, how to get erections, and other steps for men," she says, "but because women were only 20 percent or so of the SCI population, there had not been a lot of research done on us when I got hurt."

As she continued her rehabilitation, Meredith mapped out a plan. She would work on regaining the ability to do the things that were important to her—dancing, sailing, driving, working—and then think about starting a family: "I would get to a point in my life where I was happy and comfortable with myself and back to where I was when I got injured, ready to get pregnant and have a kid." That moment eventually arrived three years later. "It happened in the middle of the night," she recalls with a laugh. "I woke up my husband at three o'clock in the morning, and I said, 'I'm ready.' He said, 'Yeah, great. What for?' And I said, 'I'm ready to have a baby.'"

When Meredith asked one of her doctors what he thought about her wish to become pregnant, however, he told her that she should wait because she was taking the anti-spasticity drug Lioresal (baclofen), which is recommended against during pregnancy. He suggested that she start tapering the medication and look into alternative ways to manage her muscle tone before trying to conceive. She subsequently spent the next four months researching different options. She even considered botulinin toxin (Botox) injections to weaken the nerves in her legs until she read a medical study in which four of sixteen paralyzed women who had received such injections had miscarriages.

Next Meredith tried electrical stimulation, in which electrodes were placed on the muscles of her legs with the most spasticity. Attempting to "tire out" the muscles, she underwent this treatment with a physical therapist twice weekly to see how much her spasms could be reduced—and for how long. "Another method used to treat spasticity is a high-temperature pool," Meredith explains. "Although hot-water swimming is not really recommended for pregnant women, we wondered whether we could tire the muscles out more by combining electrical stimulation with short sessions in an 85-degree pool, which is a cooler-than-usual temperature. That combination did work, and my doctor finally gave Dylan and me the go ahead to start trying to conceive.

"Within fifteen days, we were pregnant," she continues. "I was thrilled beyond thrilled. Every woman who is having a baby feels as though there is a miracle happening inside her body. For a woman with paralysis, however, having a baby grow in the area that normally causes you nothing but angst, problems, spasticity, and incontinence was unbelievable. Nothing works correctly from my waist down, so to have this child who would end up perfectly healthy growing there was a miracle *beyond* what other women can possibly understand. Finally, this part of my body was giving me some happiness."

A NINE-MONTH CHALLENGE

The next task for the couple was finding an obstetrician who was comfortable with SCI, a process, Meredith says, that she "would not wish upon anyone." Although they finally found a doctor who dealt with high-risk pregnancies, Meredith still had concerns. "One of the things that worried me throughout the pregnancy was that if something was going wrong, I wouldn't be able to *feel* it. For me, the signs would have to be external—either by some sort of bleeding or a lack of movement that I could see or sense with my hand. I never really could tell if the baby was moving. I could feel a fullness there, and some pressure. But I couldn't experience the normal sensation."

Knowing that she was at higher risk for weight gain because

of her paralysis, Meredith was also very concerned about losing her mobility. As a result, she not only watched what she ate but also planned ahead and ordered a new wheelchair with a wider seat and less camber (wheel angle) that could accommodate the extra weight in her hips and buttocks. She also ordered it with a second axle so she could return it to her preferred seating after her pregnancy. "When sitting in a wheelchair, your hips are at the same exact level as the tires," she says. "So with the reduced camber, the wheels wouldn't lean in and hit my bigger hips; they would be more up and down—which, while harder to push, is a lot less painful. I was also very concerned about developing pressure sores from the added weight, so I just did pressure relief like crazy." In the end, Meredith gained only twenty-five pounds before she delivered, and she remained able to alternate comfortably between her new and old chair.

There were other challenges as well. During the birthing classes that she and Dylan took along with ten able-bodied couples, Meredith remembers "feeling like a square peg." Because a lot of the exercises took place on the floor, following the routines was often quite awkward for her and Dylan. Even more difficult was the severe swelling in her feet that occurred during the final month of her pregnancy. It prevented her from wearing her braces and, therefore, doing much driving. "With the extra twenty-five pounds, I could only get out of the driver's seat and get to the back of my car to grab my wheelchair once a day," she remembers. "The fatigue was incredible."

Overall, however, Meredith admits that being pregnant gave her an incredible sense of well-being. "I just felt like I was on top of the world all the time," she says. "I also really didn't have much morning sickness." Throughout her pregnancy, she continued with water therapy three times a week and electrical stimulation twice daily. When her spasticity improved significantly in the last few months (possibly due to hormonal changes), she was able to decrease the frequency of her therapy. She did continue to swim on her own, though, because "it was so good for the swelling and my well-being, and it offered some relief from the weight of the pregnancy."

LABOR AND DELIVERY

"I was nine days late, and my doctor really preferred that I have a planned delivery, either a C-section or an induction," says Meredith. "I refused. I wanted a natural birth; I wanted the baby to come when it wanted to come, and I wanted as little drug intervention as possible. Because I wasn't at risk for autonomic dysreflexia [owing to the level of her injury], I wanted to reap the benefits of the paralysis [the decreased perception of pain] and hopefully not need the type of pain medicine that other women often do."

The couple lived about an hour from the hospital where Meredith delivered, and by the time they arrived there the morning she went into labor, her contractions were two-and-a-half minutes apart. "It was like a gripping cramp on my abdomen that caused me to lose my breath," she recalls. "It was the greatest amount of discomfort I had experienced since I was paralyzed. Each contraction was like a sharp thunderbolt that made breathing difficult. I thought if I was able to feel things this much, then the baby must be coming. When I was younger, I had always been fearful of the pain associated with childbirth, but now I had gone through the pain of breaking my back. I had survived *that* intensity of pain, so I suspected that nothing could ever hurt that much again. I knew I could make it through this."

Concerned about the possibility that an obstetrician other than her own might assist with the delivery, Meredith had compiled written information describing the details of her spinal cord injury and the subsequent changes in her muscle strength and sensation that could affect her medical care. "I figured there

were very few nurses and doctors out there who had real experience with SCI, so I came prepared with a bunch of documents to
help them understand my condition," she says. "I wanted them
to know that 'I don't have some of the sensation normally relied
upon by a 'standard' woman giving birth, and I don't know how
much I'm going to feel. So if you're looking to me to tell you
how it's progressing, for example, I probably won't be able to tell
you. You're going to have to tell *me*.' In fact, that turned out to
be true."

Another reason for the documentation was to highlight certain requests that might otherwise be overlooked. "I wanted the
team to realize that I needed to be able to use my arms so that I
could move in the bed," Meredith explains. "One of the problems I'd had before in the hospital was that they would stick the
intravenous line in the inside of my elbow. With the IV there, I
was completely unable to move and position myself. They were
essentially immobilizing me. So I let them know that I preferred
the IV on the outside or inside of my forearm, or even on the
back of my hand."

Meredith's delivery turned out to be faster than expected. "We
got there at 3 A.M. and delivered the baby at 11:23," she says.
"Things didn't get intense until the last ninety minutes or so.
Just before delivering, I felt some sort of change—like a change
in blood pressure. I told the nurse that something felt different,
and I asked if she wouldn't mind checking. So she did an internal examination, and then yelled, 'I see a baby! I see hair!' Suddenly a whole team of doctors came in. Because I was seen as
sort of a guinea pig, there were all these medical residents who
wanted to see the birth. It seemed like the equivalent of a football team at the end of my bed. They all came in and put on their
gowns, and then the [lead] doctor said, 'Give me one push.' I did,
and then he said, 'Give me one more—and all you've got!' I did,
and the baby was delivered. She was born on my birthday, Feb-

ruary 25, so we're exactly thirty-five years apart in age. In the end, the experience was much easier than I had expected, and I was so surprised that it all went so well. Fifteen minutes after the birth, I turned to my husband and said, 'Let's have another.'"

Cindy and Ted

Ask Cindy Purcell if the "uneducated public" was surprised to learn that she and her husband, Ted—both of whom have tetraplegia—were expecting a baby, and she answers quickly: "Of course. Number one, people think you're not sexually capable. I mean, how can people in wheelchairs have sex? It's not normal, right? They were either amazed when I told them we *could* get pregnant, or they thought the baby was going to be born with a disability. They just didn't understand it."

CONCEPTION: PERSISTENCE PAYS OFF

Cindy and Ted were, in fact, completely capable of having a child. Cindy's ability to become pregnant was not affected by her injury, and Ted was still able to ejaculate during intercourse. Nobody who knew them doubted their ability to be great parents, but after several years of trying, they had still not been able to conceive. To improve the couple's chances, doctors recommended that Ted use a vibrator to ensure that his sperm was sufficiently potent. When this didn't work, the pair sought the assistance of a reproductive endocrinologist. Able to pinpoint the specific time each month when Cindy's fertility was at its peak, the doctor would take a sperm sample from Ted and place it into her cervix with a catheter, a process known as IUI. Cindy had to lie upside down throughout the procedure.

"It didn't work right away, and it was so hard to wait for the phone call with the results," recalls Cindy. "The first few calls the nurse just said, 'I'm sorry, Cindy, not this time.' The third time the results came back, it was Ted's birthday, October 16. My office had glass walls, so everybody outside my door was looking in when I got the call. They all knew what was going on. This time, the nurse said, 'Congratulations!' I tried not to go crazy before I called Ted. I said, 'Happy birthday, *Dad.*' Everybody cheered, and it was great."

GETTING THROUGH THE NINE MONTHS

Once she was pregnant, Cindy's biggest fear was that the accompanying weight gain might cause dysreflexia—which at times it did—and that problems like constipation would keep her from carrying the baby to term, which they did *not*. Still, she never doubted her and Ted's decision. "I was always excited about having a child," she recalls, "but there were no other SCI women I knew who had had kids—nobody to learn about the experience from." In the end she didn't gain too many pounds on her slight frame, which meant not having to worry about one of the things that veteran SCI moms, like Meredith, could have warned her about—the need for a bigger wheelchair during the third trimester. Could she feel her baby kicking inside her? "All the time," she says with a smile.

"The only problem I ever had was some bad urinary tract infections," she explains. "I would get very dysreflexic and have to go to the hospital. The funny thing was, we were friendly with all the EMTs and cops in our small town, so they knew to be on alert. One night my infection was really bad, and the cop who came in was also a part-time nurse at a local rehab hospital. He was able to check my catheter and everything. They put me on antibiotics, which was pretty tricky because they had to make sure the drugs were safe for the baby and worked for me. Everything turned out okay."

As Ted is quick to point out, Cindy is always quite modest in her recollections. She often forgets, for instance, other complications like the yeast infection that developed in her bladder during treatment for one of her upper respiratory infections. Then there were the long nights spent trying to sleep on her left side, the recommended position to optimize blood flow to the developing fetus. Cindy kept rolling over onto her back, but Ted was always there to roll her into position again. It was also during this time, Cindy recalls, that a urologist who heard about her multiple urinary tract infections "openly questioned why Ted and I were doing this [trying to get pregnant]." When this particular doctor met the couple, however, he immediately realized their capabilities and commitment to parenthood. "He wound up telling my O.B. that it was wonderful we were having a child."

THE WHOLE WORLD WATCHING—ALMOST

Although Cindy's doctor knew that her baby was in the breech position (feet first), he was hesitant to try to turn or manipulate him (as is often attempted in these situations), because the head was literally resting on Cindy's rib cage. Subsequently, a planned cesarean section was decided upon for around 32–34 weeks gestation, though it was actually performed at 38 weeks. Documenting each of these milestones was a camera crew from the ABC T.V. News show *20/20,* which the couple had agreed to let develop a segment around their pregnancy. "Our intent was to show other people with disabilities that they could have kids," explains Cindy. "Of course, not everybody with disabilities *should* have kids, just for the same reasons that not every able-bodied person should have them. Disability should never be the reason on its own."

When it came time for her delivery, Cindy opted, as many moms-to-be do, for epidural anesthesia to help with the pain. Again, this surprised people who lacked full knowledge of the couple's circumstances. "People would say to me, 'You're so lucky, you don't have to have a spinal because you can't feel your baby,' and I would have to explain that even if *I* can't feel, my *body* feels [autonomic dysreflexia]. I don't get very testy about peoples' ignorance, because sometimes people just need things explained to them—including doctors. That was something I learned when first going through rehab after my accident, and I've kept it in mind ever since. The therapists told me flat out, 'You have to know yourself and your body, because nobody else is going to know it better than you.' It's very true.

"I worked late on a Thursday, and Tanner was born the following day, June 13. We had the camera people from *20/20* and a reporter from the local newspaper in the delivery room with us, but I really didn't mind. As a little girl, I had always dreamed about being a mom, but if you brought it up soon after my accident I would have said you were crazy. Now it was happening, and everything was just perfect."

For Meredith, Cindy, and other women with spinal cord injury, having a baby can be a reality rather than a dream. With the proper medical care, paralysis should have little impact on pregnancy, labor, or delivery. Although challenges may occur along the way, many individuals have shown that with determination, preparation, and adaptability, pregnancy and motherhood is possible. And just as increasing numbers of paralyzed women are making the decision to bear children and learn more about the process, physicians are becoming more experienced in dealing with pregnancy and SCI. Like so many other aspects of life with disability, the key to having a baby—for paralyzed women and men—is to focus on what *is* possible rather than what is not.

Parenting with SCI: Moms and Dads on Wheels

After numerous outings with her newborn daughter, Meredith had come to expect the comments. "I'd be out with Dina doing errands, and a store clerk or cashier would take one look at her, one look at me in my wheelchair, and ask politely: 'Are you babysitting?' or 'Did you adopt?'" she explains. "At first I found it amusing, but eventually all the comments got me angry. I could swear that many of these same people had seen me around town during my pregnancy, but I guess they hadn't noticed my growing stomach because I was always seated."

Even if people had missed her pregnancy, Meredith notes, that certainly didn't explain why they seemed to have trouble realizing—or believing—that Dina could actually be her biological child. "People just don't expect women with disabilities to be able to give birth," she says. "They don't see us as sexual beings, therefore they don't see us as mothers. But I found a way to let out some of my frustration without being too rude. I'd look them in the eye, smile, and say, 'Yes, disabled people do have sex, they do get pregnant, and they do have babies—all by choice!'"

When Cindy Purcell's son, Tanner, was four, she received a call from his nursery school. "His teacher had overheard one of the other students telling kids in class about the time his grandmother was 'sick in a wheelchair' and needed to take an ambulance to the hospital," Cindy recalls. "The teacher was worried that Tanner might start

thinking I was sick too because I used a wheelchair, so she invited
me in to speak to the class about living with disability. Although I
had always made a conscious effort not to do anything that would
elicit sympathy or make me stand out from other parents at school
events, I accepted the offer. And in the end I was delighted with
what happened. Not only was Tanner not embarrassed by my
appearance; he was so proud that he got up and started showing
classmates how my wheelchair worked, and all the 'neat stuff' it
could do."

After Matt was paralyzed in a skiing accident just after his fortieth
birthday, he worried about how using a wheelchair would affect his
abilities as a parent. "I had coached my four kids' sports teams and
loved taking the whole family on vacations or just playing around
the house," he says. "Now I thought I'd no longer be able to enjoy
this type of active lifestyle, and that my relationship with my kids
would suffer. When I had to miss my oldest daughter's birthday
while undergoing rehabilitation at a facility 1,000 miles away, then
heard about the teasing she and her siblings had to go through once
the news about my condition had gotten around, my concerns and
frustration grew."

Looking back, Matt says that it was only by focusing on the great
family he had waiting for him after rehab that he was able to get
through those difficult first few months. He knew that he might
never walk unaided again, but he was alive—and there were plenty
of things he could still do as a father and a husband. This kind of
positive attitude helped him return to the coaching ranks and ski
slopes in just a year, and in 2004 he was named "Citizen of the
Year" in the small Massachusetts town where he and his family
reside.

Parenting is a tough job for anybody—one filled with intense
emotional and physical demands at every stage of a child's life.

The hours are long and the challenges many, but most mothers and fathers will say that the rewards are worth all the effort. The majority of individuals who take on this role have the full use of their arms and legs, but when people require the assistance of others to get dressed, move around, or use the bathroom, the responsibility of loving, nurturing, and disciplining one or more kids becomes a task more formidable than most parents can even imagine. Yet these are the circumstances under which many men and women handle life's greatest "duty" on a daily basis.

Each year spinal cord injuries leave thousands of people suddenly dependent on wheelchairs and/or personal care attendants at the same time that their children are still dependent on *them*. This combination requires extra patience and perseverance on the part of these moms and dads as they strive to maintain their parental roles. Moreover, a growing number of other couples (as well as individuals) are making the choice to conceive or adopt children *after* SCI and voluntarily open themselves up to many of the same challenges, along with the potential for negative reactions from strangers and even loved ones who believe that their decision to start a family post-injury is an irresponsible act.

It is, in fact, nothing of the sort. As the first substantial studies of children brought up by disabled parents have proven in recent years, the myth that mothers and fathers with spinal cord injuries lack the capacity to fulfill these roles is unfounded. (See Suggested Reading for specific studies.) Boys and girls raised by one or even two such parents are no less happy, healthy, or confident than kids with able-bodied moms and dads. Moreover, they have been found to be especially compassionate and open-minded about people's differences, as we might expect given their exposure to disability at an early age.

The credit goes to everybody involved. Although it may take extraordinary patience, mental energy, and planning to get through each day, these dedicated families are showing that it is possible to parent with SCI. In addition, many of them have been strong, vocal advocates for accessibility and acceptance in schools, sports leagues, and other venues, as well as leaders in forming networking groups within the SCI and general disability communities. Their refusal to let SCI keep them from experiencing life to the fullest is largely responsible for society's changing notions about what people with disabilities can and do accomplish.

This wasn't always the case. Not long ago paralyzed moms and dads like Meredith, Cindy, and Matt had few resources or peers to turn to when faced with the myriad challenges of child rearing. Before the 1980s, far fewer people with SCI chose to have kids; and when they did, they had almost no role models (or public agencies) to help them. In this way, new parenthood postinjury was just one of the many aspects of everyday life that was closed off to disabled individuals as recently as several decades ago. In fact, it's likely that many paralyzed people themselves shared the same uninformed opinion as the shop owners Meredith encountered: bearing and raising children was simply not something they were expected—or encouraged—to do. When disabled women *did* become pregnant, they were often persuaded to have abortions or to give up their children for adoption.

One reason for the lack of support at this time was the dubious research findings about the potential impact that parenting with disability could have on a child's development. Although studies on parenting with *any* kind of disability were scarce, those that were conducted were usually extremely negative in tone and based more on speculation than on fact. In analyzing this research, the disability advocates Megan Kirschbaum and Rhoda Olkin found biases at work in these studies that were often echoed in the general public's viewpoint on the subject. (Kirschbaum is founder and executive director of Through the Looking Glass, an organization and advocacy group profiled later in this chapter.)

Most of the investigations, they explained, grouped together people with various types and degrees of disability, including visual impairment and paralysis, to reach their conclusions; as a result, these findings were not applicable to any one specific group. Even parents whose disabilities were cognitive in nature were often misleadingly labeled as "parents with physical disabilities" and grouped with paralyzed mothers and fathers in various articles and studies. Another problem was that any other, co-existing factors that might contribute to difficulties raising children, including parental substance abuse and poverty, were ignored. If disability existed in troubled families, it was blamed for the dysfunction.

Moreover, at this time most research on disabled parents was focused solely on fathers—then, as now, approximately 80 percent of spinal cord injuries occurred in men—and these studies, too, painted a primarily bleak picture. One of the main theories put forth was that a father's disability would severely stress his family, thereby leading to increased emotional insecurity for the children. Having a paralyzed father was thought to threaten a child's adjustment, potentially harming his or her personality development, athletic interests, interpersonal relations, and even sexual identity. Such generalized, stereotypical opinions were not only printed as "facts" in textbooks but also used by adoption agencies and the courts to deny parental responsibilities to people with disabilities.

Dispelling the Myths

With the passage of the Americans with Disabilities Act (ADA) in 1990, many new laws were enacted to protect both paralyzed individuals and their children from discrimination in the courts and elsewhere. Additionally, numerous organizations sprang up to support these families and educate the public, which in turn led to changing attitudes about what makes someone a "capable" caregiver. Research findings during the 1990s were also much more positive in tone, revealing that more and more disabled people were seeking—and, when necessary, fighting for—the right to have children. This trend has continued into the new millennium, accompanied by a growing public acceptance of these families. Although pockets of prejudice and ignorance still exist, as do custody battles in which a parent's physical limitations are brought to the forefront, it is now widely accepted in the professional and lay communities that being disabled does not in itself preclude someone from being a good mother or father.

More recent studies have shown, for instance, that children of mothers and fathers with spinal cord injury are just as well adjusted and emotionally stable as their peers with nondisabled parents. Furthermore, no differences were noted in their sex-role development, self-esteem, or body image. One research team found that many children with paralyzed dads actually felt *more* competent and ready to face the world than those with able-bodied fathers, as a result of their daily exposure to the challenges of disability. I have heard similar thoughts from many disabled parents themselves, who are quick to point out that their own children display maturity—and sensitivity—beyond their years.

"She's very responsible, and the teachers say she's almost like a mother hen at school," says Marlene, a single mom with T10 paraplegia, of her seven-year-old daughter, Heidi. "If she sees a kid with a book having trouble reading, she'll go over and help him sound out the words. Once a girlfriend of hers was getting picked on, and she really gave it to the bully. She sticks up for the little guy, and I think that's definitely connected to my injury."

As another example, Marlene enjoys telling about the time Heidi was four and they were vacationing in Florida. "She wanted to go to

the pool, and I wasn't ready yet. So she went and invited herself to
go along with a woman we had just met who had multiple sclerosis
and was in a wheelchair. Even now when she sees a person in a
wheelchair, she's more trusting of them than of people who can
walk."

Another frequently cited concern of the past—the negative impact of a spinal cord–injured parent's physical limitations on a child's leisure-time activities—has also been shown to have little validity. For example, the paralyzed dads who were observed in an early 1980s study led by Frances Marks Buck and George Hohmann participated in as many recreational activities as other fathers, and their children were actually *more* interested in sports and similar pastimes than youngsters whose fathers didn't need a wheelchair to get around the basketball or tennis court. Other research has shown this to also be true for disabled moms on and off the fields of play. Although in previously published studies, as well as in personal interviews conducted for this book, children of those with SCI did cite challenges involved with having one or even two disabled parents, they claimed to experience no increased social stigma because of this situation. They denied being teased or "pitied"; nor did they have fewer close friends than their peers—either in earlier childhood or in adolescence. Their teenage dating patterns were also generally not affected by their parents' paralysis, and as a group, they professed to taking extra steps to involve their disabled parents in their social lives.

Moreover, research has shown that these same children regard their paralyzed parents as warm, affectionate, and playful. In a 2002 study of more than 150 families, Craig Alexander and colleagues found no significant differences between mothers with SCI and their able-bodied counterparts when it came to loving and nurturing their kids. Researchers who focused on disabled dads found similar results; Frances Marks Buck led a 1981 study, for example, in which disabled fathers were shown to be *more* physically and verbally affectionate toward their kids than able-bodied dads. Their children also reported loving, respecting, and being proud of them, and not just because these kids felt that having disabled dads allowed them to get away with more mischief.

On the contrary, when it came to discipline, fathers in this situation reported using the exact same methods as other parents, including reasoning, yelling, and even spanking. Nonetheless, Buck noted, their sons and daughters "reported significantly more positive attitudes toward their fathers than did comparison children." The earlier presumptions that disabled parents would either have to relegate all disciplinary responsibilities to their able-bodied mates or watch their children grow up with no limits or rules whatsoever have been unsupported.

According to recent literature, having a mother or father with SCI does not negatively affect children's psychological adjustment; nor does it increase stress or conflict. In reality, parental attitudes and behavior in the household, most specifically the ability to create a warm, structured environment, appear to be most vital for successful child rearing and family functioning. As many disabled moms and dads are quick to point out, there are just as many of them who *can* provide these intangibles as there are able-bodied people who *cannot* (and end up with troubled kids as a result). It is now clear that a person's ability to walk unaided has nothing to do with his or her ability to create and maintain a loving, accepting parent-child relationship.

"She can hop in my lap, sure, but I want to be able to get on the ground and not worry about throwing myself back into my wheelchair," explains Danny, a man with paraplegia, of life with his infant daughter. "I want to be able to go on the beach and build sand cas-

tles with her and feel the sand between my toes or go in the backyard and kick a soccer ball with her. I want to do tons of things that
able-bodied fathers can do and take for granted—but I can't. What
I can do is be there for her and be involved with her and have a positive influence on her. I can teach her how to play tennis and be with
her at soccer games. I can be part of a lot of activities in different ca-
pacities. It's all about how you get used to things—and how willing
you are to adapt. Life with a spinal cord injury sucks, but you can
still live a happy life—it's all about how you adapt."

Different Stages, Different Concerns

Entering Parenthood

Even with so much information supporting their capabilities as
mothers and fathers, people with SCI can still face prejudice
from the general public or in some cases even from close friends
and family. As one woman described it, parents with disabilities
are sometimes "non-visible" to the masses because people may
be unable to look past the wheelchairs or other equipment to see
them in a guardian role. Thus it is up to the individuals themselves to change these perceptions, which start as soon as they
begin discussing plans for parenthood and find their loved ones
questioning their decision. "Don't you already have enough to
handle?" is a common response. "Are you sure you want to deal
with the pressures of raising a child?" While concerns like these
might be well intentioned, they can also be hurtful to people
bearing such exciting news.

One paralyzed woman who told her mother that she could, in
fact, get pregnant and was currently trying to do so was met
with a cynical retort: "Great—you're going to get pregnant and
have a kid, and I'm the one who is going to have to take care of
it." Although the woman realized that her mother's comments

stemmed from fear rather than from selfishness, they were still hurtful. Another mother-to-be with paraplegia heard even more shocking responses from her relatives. "They said I didn't have the right to have children because I was disabled," she recalled years later. "They questioned how I could expect to have a fulfilling life when I wouldn't be able to do things for myself or for my child."

Such insensitivity and ignorance can even extend to the medical community. While some women with SCI have been able to find physicians who are prepared to deal with the special challenges their pregnancies present (see Chapter 8), others find themselves at the mercy of doctors who lack experience or an understanding of the women's situation. These doctors may not know, for instance, whether a specific medication used for morning sickness or migraines might cause complications for women with paraplegia. Thus some women seeking empathetic caregivers are left disappointed.

One woman noted that her obstetrician—who used phrases like, "For a *normal* woman the experience would be . . ."; or, "Under *normal* circumstances the delivery pain would be . . ."— could not answer the majority of her questions. Instead, he would continually defer to her rehabilitation doctor for most of her care. Although the general public is certainly better informed today than several decades ago, comments such as, "How can *you* be having a child?" can still crop up once it becomes obvious that a paralyzed woman is pregnant—unless, as in Meredith's case, no one even notices.

These kinds of uninformed comments may even continue after the child is born. Some people who see a disabled mother and a baby girl together, for instance, just assume that the infant is a granddaughter or a niece. Adopted babies who look noticeably different from their moms can also elicit inappropriate comments from strangers. One disabled Caucasian woman I know who adopted a girl from Central America was playing with her daughter in the yard one day when a neighbor exclaimed, "You two spend so much time together—she's going to start thinking you're her mother!" Recounting the incident later, the mom was not sure if the neighbor mistook her role because her skin color was different from her daughter's or because she used a wheelchair.

Given such hardships, it is not surprising that paralyzed women run an increased risk of postpartum depression. While an estimated 20 percent of *all* new mothers deal with feelings of anxiety, sadness, or apathy that persist in the months after giving birth, these emotions are known to be more common—and actually compounded—in those women who also may face the challenges of disability. Although many moms who stay at home caring for an infant can experience pangs of loneliness or "cabin fever," this challenge is even greater for individuals with paraplegia or tetraplegia who have less opportunity for (and ability to make) brief, spontaneous escapes to friends' houses or the gym. And while these disabled mothers may try to do whatever they can to prepare themselves mentally for the fact that they will need extra help with their children, they often find it much harder than they imagined to watch a relative or personal care attendant feed, clothe, or bathe their son or daughter when they are unable to do so by themselves. (For more on the danger of depression among all individuals with spinal cord injury, see Chapter 3.)

In seeking support, moms and dads can turn to fellow paralyzed parents who have encountered—and successfully met—such challenges. In addition, numerous articles and books addressing pregnancy, childbirth, and parenting with a disability have become available in recent years, though there is truly no substitute for talking with others who have firsthand experience. The problem, however, is locating these resources; in the greater Boston and western Massachusetts area, for example, only a handful of women with SCI who gave birth between 1990 and 2004 could be found four years later. As membership in this unique community increases, more people will gain access to groups and individuals who can help them through the tough spots, assisted largely by the growing number of websites and online chat rooms devoted to the subject.

Infants and Toddlers

BABIES AND THE ART OF ADAPTING

Just as with the numerous other challenges people face after spinal cord injury—including pregnancy and childbirth—many individuals and couples have successfully adapted to their new roles as parents. Despite the physical limitations and time constraints they confront from the beginning, these mothers and fathers have demonstrated considerable ingenuity in developing solutions to their childcare difficulties. Although those with higher levels of injury and less dexterity may require more physical assistance than others, they can still be active participants in their offsprings' care by remaining close by and "directing" their helpers. Accustomed to daily problem solving, people with all levels of SCI are able to apply that same creativity, determination, and resourcefulness toward parenthood. No matter what a person's physical impairments, the opportunity for powerful bonding with one's children is possible—it will just take more effort for people with SCI.

Preparation can begin well before a baby is even born. While the only training that many able-bodied future parents receive may be prenatal child-birthing classes or talking with friends or relatives, disabled people benefit from much more extensive planning. Since, for instance, the act of transporting a tiny, fragile person from room to room or across town can be daunting, some prospective moms and dads have "borrowed" the babies of relatives or friends to practice and thereby increase their confidence. By learning in advance what is and isn't possible, they are then able to take the necessary steps to prepare for their own future arrival.

Meredith recalls that getting her young daughter in and out of cars before the toddler could walk was "the hardest part of being a wheelchair mom" because the task put so much weight on her lower back and required strong trunk balance. Having the chance to perfect this maneuver before Dina was born, she attests, proved invaluable. "I didn't want to have the baby and then find out I couldn't go anywhere," Meredith recalls of her pregnancy. "I was terrified of that happening, so I wanted to get all of my fears and possible problems out of the way. One friend would come over with her car, another with her kid, and I'd work with them both. People were so willing to help me figure these things out ahead of time that it really put me at ease.

"I bought a car seat with the lowest possible sides—the most open-faced car seat you can get with the smallest barrier between you and the baby. A baby carrier that I wore on my chest was my No. 1 piece of essential equipment. The only way I could transfer to a wheelchair with Dina in the beginning was to have her in this carrier. That was how I got her from Point A to Point B on an everyday basis; a "regular" mom could just throw a kid on her hip to carry her back and forth. I basically had to carry Dina to the car door in the carrier, and then pitch her like a football into the car seat."

HELPING HANDS

No amount of preparation can ready a new mother or father for the powerful flood of emotions that accompanies the birth of a baby. For parents with the most severe disabilities, however, these traditional feelings of joy and nervousness may be accompanied by a sense of remorse when they realize that they cannot tend to many of their new infants' needs on their own. One paralyzed mother, describing her feelings in the first days of her baby's life, stated, "I was heartbroken when my daughter cried and could only be comforted by someone else while I just looked on. The people who were 'helping' me were unknowingly taking my role as my baby's mother, because only they could ensure that my child's needs were being met. If family and well-meaning friends just take over, they aren't really helping."

What this woman and many disabled parents eventually come to realize is that even if you aren't the person holding, dressing, or feeding your child, you can still have a significant presence in his or her daily life. Whether it means picking out an outfit, deciding when to offer a bath or bottle, or simply sitting nearby and chatting with a son or daughter while others change a diaper or cook a meal, such contributions can make a parent feel more actively involved. While disabled mothers and fathers have every reason to feel proud about what they are able to do by themselves with their children, there is no shame in seeking help through a personal care attendant or other means. Parents should remember two important things: they are ultimately the ones in charge of any decisions regarding their children, and if they find that they don't like what a PCA or another assistant is doing, they are always free to find someone else.

One program, the Toronto-based Nurturing Assistance service, originated when a mother who was disabled required help after her first child was born in 1988. This program provides physical assistance to disabled parents with children up to ten years old, by supplying help with whatever day-to-day tasks are necessary, including bathing, changing diapers, preparing meals, even cuddling. Although parents must pay for these nurturing assistants and are still responsible for the health and safety of their children, the support provided is often priceless. In many ways, these helpers are like "bonus" personal care attendants, relieving disabled mothers and fathers of some of their physical duties, and thereby giving them extra time and energy to focus on their emotional bonds with their children. Those who have employed nurturing assistants admit to experiencing a greater sense of dignity and control over their households and lives. In fact, several additional agencies have subsequently been set up to help families pay for the assistants, and the Centre for Independent Living in Toronto (CILT) has even published a how-to book for families and service providers that details ways to develop and best benefit from this program.

THE PARENT'S CHAMPION: THROUGH THE LOOKING GLASS

Another support system available for disabled parents as they prepare for and start to raise their children is Through the Looking Glass (or TLG), a Berkeley-based nonprofit organization founded in 1982 by the infant/family therapist Megan Kirschbaum. Initially based in a garage and funded with a $5,000 grant from the March of Dimes, TLG has grown into an internationally recognized group that employs psychologists, occupational therapists, rehabilitation counselors, family therapists, and other experts focused on ensuring that no family is denied the opportunity to thrive despite disability. The organization has conducted pioneering research into parenting with disabilities, developed innovative therapy techniques, and designed various assistive baby care equipment for disabled mothers and fathers, while also teaching them how to adapt their own gear.

Not surprisingly, Through the Looking Glass has emerged as a leading voice in the disability movement. In 1998 it received a five-year grant from the National Institute on Disability and Rehabilitation Research (NIDRR) and the United States Department of Education to form the National Resource Center for Parents with Disabilities, which provides information, referrals, publications, training, and consultations on parenting. A National Task Force Report put out by TLG the same year recommended that, despite the gains that have been made since the

ADA was passed nearly a decade before (in 1990), there was still a need to improve conditions for disabled parents and their children. The task force described the need to increase available options for and access to childcare; to provide accessible and adequate housing and transportation options; and to increase public awareness in order to reduce attitudinal barriers.

Through the Looking Glass aims to give people with disabilities the information and empowerment they need to be more effective parents, as well as to better enjoy the experience of raising kids. The organization's National Parent-to-Parent Network (which was also established through the 1998 NIDRR grant) connects prospective or newly disabled parents with "veterans" who can teach what they've learned from years of experience. In this way, moms and dads worldwide are able to gain support as they work through challenges—both those unique to their situation and those faced by *all* families. By improving the childrearing experience, Kirschbaum and her staff have helped countless people with disabilities enjoy a part of life once largely closed off to them. The organization's website (http:// lookingglass.org) says it best: "The connotation of our name is that the disability experience does not have to be just negative or traumatic. Like Alice's *Through the Looking Glass* experience, disability brings new perspectives that can engender creativity and new meanings—even playfulness and humor! The reflection of the looking glass also points to the profound role people who have been through this process can play for one another."

BABY EQUIPMENT

The success of Through the Looking Glass is in many ways directly linked to the frustration that many paralyzed moms and dads feel on making their first trip to the baby superstore and discovering that most infant paraphernalia is not designed with them in mind. Nearly all cribs and bassinets are either too high or too low for a person who has difficulty bending down or standing up to reach a baby, and dropside-style cribs, with sides designed to pull in and then down for easy access to the infant, are usually too complicated for someone with weak hands to manipulate. Changing tables are equally challenging, since they are also intended to be used from a standing position and are frequently equipped with several drawers underneath that, though convenient for storage, prevent wheelchair access.

Given these limitations, some paralyzed parents resort to diapering their infants on the bed, and subsequently put themselves at risk for back strain from all the forward bending required. Many are unable to accomplish the task of diapering at all because of inadequate trunk control. With few other options, many parents in this predicament choose to adapt available equipment at home to compensate for the lack of commercially available adaptive gear. Examples of this creative approach include some of the methods that manual wheelchair users have come up with to tackle the diaper-changing challenge. For instance, some have used a commercially available pad with an added safety strap atop a standard card table to create an accessible changing area, while others have adapted computer desks by removing the keyboard shelves. Either arrangement allows a wheelchair to roll underneath and puts a parent in close, safe contact with his or her infant. Once at the table, a parent can make the process of dressing a child easier by adding Velcro closures to infant shirts and pants or avoiding clothing with fasteners altogether and instead using larger-sized pullover shirts with wide scoop necks and pants with loose elastic waists.

Another concern for disabled parents is the ability to move a child around the house safely and efficiently. Moms and dads who use manual wheelchairs need their hands for maneuvering and so cannot easily carry an infant at the same time. The various commercially available sling-like baby carriers or backpacks that support a baby and don't require the use of arms would

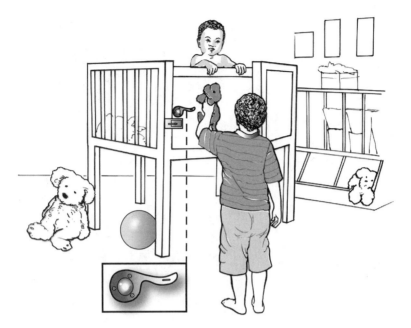

FIGURE 7.   Parents who use wheelchairs can enjoy safe, easy access to their babies and toddlers using equipment like this play/care center, constructed of wood and featuring an adaptive door handle for caregivers with limited hand function.

seem a perfect solution, but it's often difficult for people with weak hands to put their infants into them. As a result, some parents have used nursing pillows to secure their children on their laps for holding and transporting. An elastic wrist strap can be added to help position a pillow properly and keep it close, while an extra-long seat belt attachment can help ensure that little ones stay safe.

Through the Looking Glass has also been instrumental in helping develop and produce such equipment, as well as in studying its impact on parenting. The organization has published and updated an *Ideabook on Adaptive Parenting Aids,* which is filled

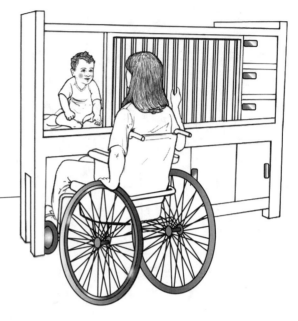

FIGURE 8.   This full side-away crib enables parents to easily place or pick up a child using a gate that smoothly rolls open and closed along a secure track. Both the crib and the play center (Figure 7) were designed by Through the Looking Glass, a nationally recognized organization helping families with disabilities.

with various devices ranging from specialized baby carriers to innovative play centers (see Figure 7). More specifically, for example, the "full side-away" crib (see Figure 8) was designed to overcome difficulties that wheelchair users have in lifting babies out of cribs or opening dropside gates. With this model, a disabled parent is able to swing the side gate open and help the infant in and out. The sliding mechanism also enables the parent to be physically close to his or her child whether the crib is open or closed.

In addition, to help with feeding, parents with weak grasps

can use a "bottle wrap" device made from webbing material and Velcro to help secure the bottle. Those who desire face-to-face contact while moving their infant about can use a baby seat attachment for power wheelchairs (see Figure 9). This device consists of a car seat attached to a metal rod with a swiveling mechanism, which is then secured to the wheelchair frame. It allows a baby to be close to the parent and face him or her when being transported, fed, or otherwise cared for.

Many individuals with spinal cord injury have found that this kind of adaptive baby care equipment greatly enhances their parent-infant interactions. It gives them more confidence in their abilities and enables them to take a more active role in the caregiving process. Moreover, the increased physical contact that such gear makes possible improves the parent-child bonding experience. Disabled moms and dads can now enjoy their kids without constantly worrying about the logistics of care. They need less help from paid assistants or family members, are less fatigued, and have more time for focused, fun activities. Their *own* physical health benefits, since the equipment helps reduce back and other musculoskeletal injuries. And, perhaps most important, adaptive gear can decrease their anxiety about the safety of their children during baby care.

Disabled parents have benefited not only from special equipment but also from adaptive baby care techniques. Through the Looking Glass's "Parent-to-Parent Network" has gathered information on alternative ways of transferring, diapering, and dressing infants that help reduce the demands of baby care and make it more efficient and satisfying. For example, to ease the task of burping an infant, the group recommends a method called "sit and lean" that incorporates the use of a fanny pack equipped with a seat support for the baby. In this approach, a parent holds the baby on his or her lap with the infant's back against mom or dad's chest. The parent then leans forward, tilt-

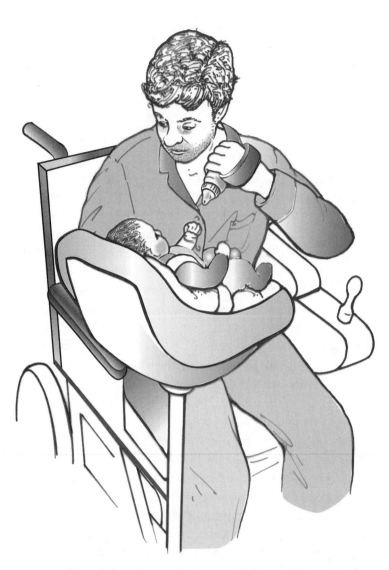

FIGURE 9.   New dads with tetraplegia can still share in feeding duties by using these two devices: a Velcro wrap that secures a bottle in one's hand, and an attachment system that fits on a power wheelchair and allows a baby to be kept safe and close.

ing the baby and increasing pressure on its stomach, resulting (hopefully) in a burp.

By making routine childcare easier for disabled parents, Through the Looking Glass has helped dispel the myth that parenting with SCI is not possible or safe. The organization stresses that the physical environment, *not* a person's physical limitations, represents the greatest barrier to childcare. Even the simplest modifications have empowered many moms and dads to go from being "passive observers" to the primary participants in their child's caregiving.

Toddlers and Young Children: Keen Learners

Disabled parents are not the only ones who have the ability to adapt creatively to childrearing. Their offspring must also learn early on to be more independent and flexible than most of their peers. Because they often assist their parents in meeting *their* needs, many of these children develop a resourcefulness beyond their years. Such adaptability will often result in a great sense of pride, not to mention excellent problem-solving skills. Whereas it was once thought that disabled parents would demand or require *so much* assistance from their children as to result in psychosocial damage to their young ones (a process known as parentification), research and interviews now indicate that this is not the case.

Tanner Purcell, the son of two parents with tetraplegia, was able to follow complex directions before he was out of diapers—partly out of a desire to help his mom and dad and partly as a result of watching personal care attendants assist his mother, Cindy, in her daily tasks. For example, by the time he was one-and-a-half, he already knew how to undo and clean his mom's leg bag, and he welcomed the chance to help with it. While Cindy's friends were hearing the famil-

iar refrain 'I can't do it, Mommy!' from their toddlers and preschool-
ers, Tanner had learned early on that he could do many of the
things that his parents couldn't do for him.

Many toddlers in this situation—and even babies—seem intu-
itively to develop more patience and tolerance for the additional
time it takes grownups with limited hand function to set up a toy
or prepare a meal. In some cases, a child may develop his or
her own "shortcuts" to compensate for parental impairments. A
daughter may discover, for example, that the easiest way to get
off Dad's lap while he's in his wheelchair is to turn on her stomach and slide feet first down to the floor, rather than have Dad
struggle with the transfer. Some disabled parents use a signal,
like quietly saying a child's name or touching his or her back, to
help their kids anticipate lifts and positional changes. After receiving such hints, my patients tell me, their toddlers will lie still
a little longer to give their parents extra time to maneuver them.
In much the same way, infants can assist parents with diapering
duties on the changing table by lifting up their bottoms. Here
again, the use of verbal or tactile cues is often helpful.

Given this added attention and "training," it is not surprising
that many kids raised under these circumstances develop certain
skills more quickly and confidently than their peers.

Meredith's daughter, Dina, learned to buckle her own car seat by
age one, after she saw how difficult the task was for her mother. In
addition, when Meredith would use her "football toss" method (ex-
plained earlier) to get Dina into the car, the toddler would make the
process easier by staying still. "Even now, years later, I still consider
the whole car seat thing to be a big deal every single time. She has
to do the buckling for me; I physically can't do it unless I go to the
other side of the car, transfer in, and sit next to her. The thing I find
so amazing is that my daughter has been buckling her own car seat

with me for years, but if an able-bodied mom helps me out by putting her in the car, Dina puts her hands on her lap and looks up as if
she's saying, 'Are you going to buckle me?' She makes the able-bodied people do it."

It's not just in the car that Dina excelled at an early age. "She
held her head up faster than any other kid, and she had trunk stability faster than any other kid," Meredith recalls. "When I went to
pick her up out of the crib—always one-handed—she would stiffen
up her whole body so I could get around her with one arm. Kids in
this situation realize what the parent needs, and they try to give it.
Dina learned to ride in a wheelchair from Day One. She was this little tiny thing; I basically would cave in my chest and put her between my breasts to get stability. I would go up the ramp and
around corners, and within a couple of days she had started to tilt to
the side to keep us from falling over. Dina had to achieve balance,
so she did.

"She's adaptable—that's the big thing," Meredith continues.
"Whereas other kids need extra time to adjust, she just acclimates to
the situation, whether it's entering a roomful of adults in a store environment or anything else. I think that adaptability comes from
having a wheelchair mom. And I think her balance and stability and
athleticism are also a result of needing to not be a blob." Other disabled parents make similar observations about their kids, including
one mom who states: "What I've found, over the years, is that my
daughters are incredibly resourceful, adaptable, and safety-conscious
because they know that I can't rescue them like other parents can.
I've noticed that able-bodied parents are very protective of their children. I can't be, so my children have become very good at self-man-
aging. They understand—at a level far beyond other children—that
if they take a physical risk, they're on their own."

In some cases, even when children are not fully able to help
their disabled parents, they may still display exceptional re-

sourcefulness. One woman with a lower lumbar spinal cord injury who could walk with braces and crutches recalled the frightening experience of slipping while walking her three-year-old
son to preschool one icy morning, and the fear that set in when
she realized she couldn't get up. Her son immediately said, "I'll
help you up, Mommy," though he lacked the strength to do so.
Snowbanks largely hid the pair from the passing cars, and nobody was in sight on the sidewalk. When the woman suggested
to her son that he run ahead to the school and get assistance, he
replied that he would never be able to open the school door on
his own. He could, however, feverishly wave his arms while his
mom did the same, and eventually they attracted the attention
of a Good Samaritan driving by. This stranger stopped and managed to assist the mother to her feet. While the boy was initially
distressed that *he* wasn't the one who had come to his mom's
rescue, he did find solace in telling her he'd be sure to do so
"when I'm big."

*Drew, who has C6-C7 tetraplegia, has a tale to share about his two-
year-old son, Artie, and seven-year-old daughter, Allison. "My grip is
poor, and Artie instinctively knows when he gives me something to
leave his hand in mine just a little bit longer to make sure I can grab
it. It's so slight other people wouldn't even notice it, but I can tell.
My kids help me all the time. If I say to Allison, 'Can I borrow your
fingers?' she knows I need help buttoning my shirt or cuffs or reaching for something. She'll make coffee for me in the morning and
does well following various directions and steps.*

*"Because Allie helps out and is incredible with her brother and
me, I can stay alone with both of them," he adds. "My wife, Angie,
will go out and leave us at home, and we can even handle Artie's diapers. I couldn't change a diaper myself, but Allison takes off the diaper, I wipe, and she puts a new one back on. When my wife*

changes Artie, he's squirming all over. But when I help change him, he's learned to be still. Also, Allison could get herself in and out of her car seat when she was sixteen or eighteen months old. Once when she was four or five, she picked up a couple of her biggest books and said, 'I'm going to find a cure for you, Daddy.' She hasn't found it yet, but she's still trying."

GETTING THROUGH THE TOUGH SPOTS

In addition to adjusting to the fact that they may never walk again, newly paralyzed parents must help their children learn to cope with the situation. This is a difficult task at any time, but it can be particularly arduous if the children are still very young.

After her accident, Marlene was initially told that she might die—a fact that she felt she had to pass on to her then three-year-old daughter Heidi. The little girl was understandably scared and a little standoffish; though Marlene recovered, the two would again be separated when Mom was transferred to a rehab facility nearly 1,000 miles away.

Two months later, Heidi was able to visit, and Marlene was nervous about seeing her. "I was scared," she recalled later. "I had still never said, 'Mommy is in a wheelchair,' so I made sure I was sitting up in bed and that she didn't see the chair right away. I was a disaster emotionally, but she was fine. The moment she saw me, she just came over and gave me a big hug. Then when I got the chair out to show her, she loved it—and loved getting a ride. She got to see that Mommy could do some of the things I used to do. I don't think we ever had a conversation about the fact that I wasn't going to walk again. She was very accepting; kids are just more resilient than we are."

More struggles ensued, however, when Marlene returned home after rehabilitation. "Heidi was very angry and used to kick me in the back," says Marlene. "She was mad all the time. If I ever said 'no' to anything she said, she'd take it out on me. I had to put her into therapy, and there they explained to me that she was really mad at the situation, not at me. Once I understood this, it was easier for me to control my temper.

"When Heidi was five and six, I was in and out of hospitals several times with pulmonary embolisms and other complications that kept me away from her for something like three months combined. She couldn't visit me much because it was too stressful for her, so I did everything I could to make sure she didn't have to worry about anything. If she was with a babysitter, I wrote up lists so that every minute of her day was documented. When she had to stay at someone else's house, I made sure it was with people who could give her lots of hugs and kisses, keep her busy, and be honest with her about the fact that I was sick."

Another way that Marlene tried—and continues trying—to make things run smoothly with Heidi is by limiting the amount of responsibility she places on her young daughter's shoulders. "I try not to ask her to help me a lot because I don't want her to feel like my caregiver," she says. "I still cook and clean and go to the grocery store, and I have a girlfriend who comes in once a week for a few hours to do heavy cleaning and run other errands. I volunteer at Heidi's school now, and one day she told me I was her hero because I feed her and love her and go to her school all the time—but not because I'm in a wheelchair."

In Marlene's view, the car accident that nearly killed her and ended her career as a paramedic and firefighter has positively affected her relationship with her daughter. "I think we're much closer than we would have been if I wasn't injured and still working sixty to eighty hours a week," she says. "Now I'm there right when she gets off the bus. Sure, I can't do the things with her that my mom and dad did with me, but I have friends who can take her. If she wants to go bike riding or swimming in a pool that's inaccessible, for in-

stance, I'll call other people to help out. As long as I can go along and share the experience with her, or she can go with somebody else she likes, that's the important thing. Every once in a while if she sees an old picture or video she'll say, 'I remember when you could walk' or 'I wish you could walk again,' but those times are few and far between. Neither of us dwells on it; it's just the way life is."

The sensitivity and acceptance exhibited by so many children of disabled parents lasts into adulthood. In fact, studies have shown that, because of the unique perspective they gain as children, many of them grow up with a heightened social consciousness, increased self-sufficiency, and tolerance for differences in others. Accordingly, they are more apt to choose "helping" professions like medicine or social work as careers.

Danny, whose young daughter has only known her dad in a wheelchair, is optimistic that the situation will have a positive impact on her development. "I hope being around me and seeing the type of person I am will give her a certain level of sensitivity to people who are 'different,' he says. "Hopefully she'll learn from me that you can't understand everybody's differences, but you need to be able to appreciate difference itself. There is a big divide between understanding and appreciating. If you take the time to ask questions and be sensitive to people who are different, that will also aid you in appreciating difference."

For children like Danny's daughter, whose parents were injured before their birth, having moms and dads who use wheelchairs isn't unusual or scary—it's all they've ever known. Creative kids quickly learn to put these contraptions to good use, for example, by grabbing the spokes of wheels to pull themselves upright when they're learning to stand or by hitching rides when they are too tired to crawl or walk.

*At the age of just three and a half, Tanner Purcell devised yet an-
other "supportive" function for his mother's wheelchair after one of
the training wheels fell off his bicycle. After finding a wrench and
taking the other training wheel off himself, he brought the bike out
onto the lawn and asked his mother to teach him to ride. With Tanner balancing the bike against the side of her chair, Cindy held it
from the back and helped glide him along. After three days, he was
riding on his own with no more help from mom. Tanner's intense
drive to succeed proved to be an early indicator of his passion for
sports. He's developed a love of baseball and basketball, and dad
Ted has coached him in both sports—from his wheelchair.*

In some cases, young children who see one or both parents
moving about on wheels may readily accept chairs as a common mode of human transport. When John Hockenberry—the
TV newsman and best-selling author who was paralyzed in college—was asked about his experience parenting four young children, he described in colorful detail how his twin daughters
learned to walk: "You could see that from their perspective, walking and the chair were two equal and interchangeable modes of
transportation. Mommy walks and Daddy uses a wheelchair.
They clearly didn't see the choice as odd or one as less than the
other."

In the end, as he wrote himself, the two infants took different
approaches to the situation: "Olivia made especially good use of
her hands and arms, grabbing tables, drawer handles, and the
spokes on my wheelchair to pull herself upright, where she
would stand in place for long periods of time, feeling the potential in her chubby little legs. Zoe . . . did not see her legs as helpful. . . . One morning . . . long before she walked, I placed Zoe in
my wheelchair and watched as she immediately grabbed the
wheels and began to push herself forward as though she'd been
doing it for years. She had even figured out how to use the dif-

ferent rotation rates of the rear wheels to steer herself. Zoe had grasped that the wheelchair was the most accessible motion platform for someone—in this case, an infant—who couldn't use her legs. She smiled as she looked at me, with an expression that said something like, 'Give up the wheels, Mr. Chairhog.'"

From his own experiences navigating around his home, Hockenberry had another reminder for fellow parents on wheels: "Little toys and little blocks will turn your accessible house into an obstacle course. You get up in the night and try and get something and suddenly you're hearing weird sounds from the toys you're running over. You're much more likely to hit one than someone walking around. Wooden blocks are the worst. They are indestructible. You'll be rolling around and they'll shut you right down."

Rhoda Olkin is another disabled author who has used her own experience to enlighten others. In her 1999 book, *What Psychotherapists Should Know about Disability*, she provides an excellent summary of what she feels are the most important attitudinal, physical, and legal barriers facing parents with disabilities. Although Olkin does not speak specifically about spinal cord injury, many paralyzed parents interviewed for this book echo her sentiments. Here are some of her observations about parenting with disability; they include both challenges and advantages:

1. Everything takes longer. Olkin believes that disability may actually *enhance* parent-child relationships by allowing families to enjoy extended intimate moments together.
2. Parents with disabilities need to rely on words to set limits for their children, discipline them, and help them with disability-related issues. Olkin and other disabled parents agree that kids whose parents can't physically "chase" them learn more quickly and at a younger age not to run off.
3. The role of adaptive equipment for parents with disabili-

ties cannot be overemphasized. Such gadgets, discussed earlier in this chapter, can help eliminate all sorts of physical and emotional barriers for families and subsequently ease childcare.

4. Moms and dads can design a style of parenting to accommodate their own disabilities. This step, of course, does not prevent disabled parents from feeling the pressure to ensure that their children are as "perfect" as possible to avoid facing prejudicial or judgmental behavior.

5. Parents with disabilities will most likely not be able to take their children to as many after-school activities as their able-bodied counterparts. Especially as these mothers and fathers age, they may not have the stamina to keep up with all the demands of today's schedule-filled youngsters.

6. At some point children will imitate a parent's disability, for example, by pretending that they can't walk or use their arms. This is not a malicious act but rather an attempt by kids to identify with their moms and dads.

7. As grownups, the children of parents with disabilities may connect with other such grown children. In addition, many become advocates for disabled people or go into other healthcare-related fields.

8. Parents with a disability often note that their children seem to take the disability as a matter of course. From the infants who learn how to scoot up onto Mom or Dad's wheelchair, to the Little Leaguers who proudly watch their folks rolling onto fields as coaches, to the teenagers who yell at them as if their only disability were being over age thirty-five, it's clear that for these kids, their parents are the same whether or not they can walk.

9. All parents seem to come equipped with a readiness to feel guilty when it comes to their children. In most cases, Olkin and others have found that such feelings are un-

warranted. As noted, most kids don't feel embarrassed or short-changed as a result of their parents' paralysis.

10. Although a parent with a disability may request assistance in performing some tasks, the generational hierarchy of parent and child—whereby the parent provides love, care, and guidance—remains intact. This fact is borne out in the research studies, described earlier in this chapter, which show that children maintain love and respect for their parents long after a mother or father's injury.

11. For all its difficulties, being a parent with a disability brings with it the same joys and rewards that having children brings to any parent. This fact, too, is validated by the comments of many interviewees who either experienced injuries after their children were born or chose consciously to have or adopt children after being paralyzed. As Olkin states, "Babies are born with a propensity to love their parents; disability does not impede this imprinting."

This list touches on both the challenges facing disabled parents, as well as the benefits that many of them experience despite the hurdles. As their children move into adolescence and young adulthood, however, they frequently seek to take on more responsibilities and freedom. Next we'll explore how their disabled moms and dads can prepare for this phase of maturity.

Older Children and Teenagers

THE STRUGGLE FOR INDEPENDENCE

As children age and begin to understand more about their parents' disabilities, new challenges—and new adjustments—arise for both parties. Whereas the physical tasks of parenting often provide the biggest struggles for spinal cord–injured individuals with babies and younger children, the barriers become more psychological in nature with older kids. Because these sons and daughters are often more independent than their peers from the beginning, they may develop even stronger urges to establish control over their lives as they age than children of able-bodied parents. By the teenage years—and sometimes earlier—the self-sufficiency that was once so helpful to their moms and dads may now become a source of tension in the home. Since these kids know that their parents cannot physically stop them from leaving the house, for instance, they may be more tempted to do so, especially if egged on by friends. Taking into account the power of peer pressure, it's crucial for paralyzed moms and dads to stick by their roles as loving guardians whose rules should be followed—even if from a wheelchair.

Just as with younger kids, issues between parents with SCI and their older offspring may differ depending on whether the paralysis occurred before or after the children were born. For those old enough to remember and comprehend the severity of a mother or father's injury when it happens, fear is a natural early reaction.

Matt's four kids—who at the time ranged in age from six to eleven—were understandably frightened when their dad was left paralyzed in a 2001 ski accident. What made the first few months he was away at rehab even more difficult were the rumors and teasing that each of them encountered at school. While many of their friends were supportive, they also heard comments like, "I heard your dad is going to die" and "Your dad is never going to be able to do anything with you again." Then there were the numerous questions from well-meaning classmates and teachers, queries they often didn't know how to answer. Daughter Elizabeth, then nine, recalls: "I felt scared, like my whole life would be different," while six-year-old Peter worried that "Dad wouldn't ever be able to play with us again." Looking back, Matt says that he and his wife could probably have helped soothe the situation in those early days by talking more openly as a family about the kids' concerns and the extent of his injuries. "We should have told them more," he says. "We'd certainly do it differently knowing what we do now."

Such levelheaded thinking is anything but easy amid the dramatic changes that can occur in the months immediately after a parent is injured. Children may have to adjust to a whole new neighborhood and school, or learn to live in a house with major physical modifications. If the paralyzed parent is temporarily or permanently unable to work, the financial ramifications can mean a significant lifestyle change (including fewer vacations, nights out, and so on). In some cases, the children's primary caregiver may change, as when an injured father stays home while Mom goes back to work. Then, of course, there are the physical changes to the individual known as "Mom" or "Dad."

One man who had several children ranging in age from preschoolers to teenagers when he became paralyzed described himself as having gone from a dad who taught by example to one who instead relied on being a communicator. "Dad still gets in the yard and throws with us. He just can't show us how to do some things," one high-schooler explained of her father. "At softball practice, as our coach, he would have to try to talk us through something, like how to stand at the plate when batting. We wouldn't understand, and he would have to get someone to show us. He gets aggravated at that."

Given the many changes that take place post-injury, it is helpful for a family to try to maintain as many of its old routines as possible—like beach trips, barbecues, and game nights. Some things simply *can't* be the same as they were before, however, and this may create frustrations for kids and parents alike. Maintaining honest, open communication among family members

allows older kids the opportunity to talk through such disappointments and more easily accept the things their parent (or
parents) can no longer do.

Kids also express appreciation for the steps their disabled parents take to remain as active as possible in their lives. When a
group of eight adolescent children who each had an injured parent were interviewed, they offered numerous examples of how
their mothers and fathers made such efforts. Even in situations
that might normally mortify teens, the warmth of the parental
gestures were very important. "There was a time when Dad's
van broke down and he wanted to get to my ballgame," one of
these interviewees recalled. "So he and my sisters borrowed a
friend's pick-up truck with a lift in the back. I'm warming up in
the outfield and see my dad riding down the street in the back of
the truck. Emily and Beth, riding in front, kept ducking down so
friends wouldn't see them. Dad is waving to everyone. He wasn't
embarrassed!"

As childhood turns to adolescence, alas, disabled parents who
have enjoyed letting their children help them with tasks may see
the frequency of this activity decrease. Whereas younger kids
may thrive on the "grownup" feeling they get from assisting
Mom and Dad, teenagers frequently become bored or even resentful of this job if it goes on for too long. Although the practice
does teach kids the value of helping others and appreciating
what they have, the pressure on sons and daughters to fulfill a
greater share of such responsibilities in families who can't afford
personal care attendants can lead to bitter feelings. (These emotions can be similar to those experienced by some couples in
which spouses serve as primary caregivers for their paralyzed
mates.)

In general, regardless of physical limitations, a parent with
spinal cord injury should be careful not to jeopardize his or her
parental role because of the need for assistance with eating,

washing up, or going to the bathroom. As one paralyzed father of six kids declared, "It's hard one minute to draw the line with the kids, and the next minute to say to the older ones, 'Oh, by the way, can you put me to bed?' It's not necessarily bad because it equalizes things, but it sometimes does make disciplining the kids a bit different."

Even the healthiest parent-child relationships often change during the teenage years. Much of this, of course, has nothing to do with a mother or father's disability. As kids become adolescents, *all* parents have a tendency to become the most embarrassing people on earth, to be avoided at all costs—especially when peers are around. Thankfully, this attitude eventually comes full circle in most cases, and parents are welcomed back into the fold by the end of college. Come adulthood, most sons and daughters are able once again to appreciate and accept their parents for who they are, wheelchairs and all.

"I see my dad as the same guy he was before," high school freshman Maddie says of her father, Matt. "I'm proud of everything he can do, but while it was cool at first when people made a big deal about him coaching our teams in a wheelchair, it's getting a little old. I don't want him or us to be treated any differently." Such feelings are right in line with Matt's own thoughts on what his injury has meant to his four children: "I think it's taught them that they can do anything. They still whine and complain like all kids, but nobody gets away with saying 'I can't' in our house. If you fall off the bike, you need to get right back on."

Children and Adolescents with SCI: The Next Generation

Jayne was the only fourth-grader at her school in a wheelchair. She had become paralyzed in a car accident when she was eight, and two years later she had only limited use of her hands and arms. In the classroom she sat at a specially designed desk that could accommodate her wheelchair, and she was able to write using a universal cuff, a special splint that held her pencil in place. When she returned to school after her accident, classmates—even those who knew her before her accident—would sometimes stare at her wheelchair. Once they got used to seeing somebody "different" in the halls, however, most of the staring stopped. Jayne eventually became friendly with a group of kids with whom she played after school.

Today, though an aide helps her catheterize her bladder in one of the building's fully accessible bathrooms, Jayne—now ten—still keeps an extra pair of underwear in her cubby just in case she has an accident. Since pressure sores are always a concern, her wristwatch has a little alarm that reminds her each fifteen minutes to shift her body weight to prevent any skin breakdown. During recess, the gym teacher helps her find special ways to participate, like giving her a large plastic bat that she can use during kickball games. "I know I can't do all the same stuff as other kids, but everybody helps me do whatever I can," Jayne says. "If I'm not feeling well or have an accident I can go right to the nurse's office without even asking my teacher, and I have a signal I give my friends so they won't worry *about me. What makes school the most fun is that most of the time, the teachers just treat me the same as everybody else."*

Justin had been swimming in the same neighbor's pool for seven years without incident, but one late June afternoon when he was thirteen, he dove in and hit his head on the pool's concrete bottom. He sustained a burst fracture of the fifth cervical vertebra and became paralyzed at the C5-C6 level. He was able to move only his wrists and elbows.

"Because I hit my head, I don't remember anything about the accident or the hours leading up to it," he says. "The first thing I do remember is being in the hospital about ten days later, which isn't so bad because it means I don't have to keep reliving the accident over and over or the first few days when I was hooked up to a respirator. There was this girl I liked, and we were kind of dating, but after she heard about what happened she never came to see me and just called one time. My friends and family were always there for me, though, both when I went home and when I went back to school."

Although certainly the most drastic, Justin's spinal cord injury was not the only major change happening to him over the next two years. He was also going through puberty, growing from 5-foot-1 and 130 pounds to 5-foot-9, 180, with a distinctly huskier voice. In the months after his return home from the rehab hospital, he struggled with not being able to go out with his friends as often or to as many places as before. He did, however, start a serious relationship with the cousin of someone he knew from rehab; because she understood a lot about paralysis, he felt comfortable discussing both his fears and his triumphs with her. His brain injury made school more of a challenge, and the former straight "A" student had to, as he explained, "relearn what I knew and use my memory in new ways." And though he had to scrap his dreams of playing football or baseball in high school, Justin managed to stay positive by sticking to the

same advice he now offers newly injured teens as a peer advisor:
"Don't be negative. Keep pushing. Never slack off. And most impor-
tantly, keep your head up."

Of the approximately 11,000 people who experience traumatic
spinal cord injuries each year in the United States, around 20
percent are under the age of twenty. The majority of this subset
of new cases are the result of motor vehicle accidents and involve older teens. Other causes of paralysis among young people
include diving, skiing, football, cheerleading, and other sports
mishaps, as well as falls. A disturbing trend in recent years has
been a growth in injuries experienced by teenagers and even
younger children as a result of violence, particularly gunshot
wounds, which disproportionately affect young men of color living in urban areas.

Not accounted for in these statistics are children whose SCI is
caused by a condition that is congenital (present at birth), such
as spina bifida, or those who become paralyzed as a result of
other nontraumatic causes that occur *after* birth, like spinal tumors, infections, and other medical conditions. While rehabilitation for people with nontraumatic SCI basically follows the
same course as treatment for individuals with traumatic injuries, children who are born with paralysis and have never known
life *without* it present their own unique set of strengths and challenges for medical personnel and loved ones.

Growing Pains

Different Ages, Different Concerns

Just as the sociological disparities between children and adults
can influence the ways these two groups become injured, physical development can have a significant impact on post-SCI com-

plications. Kids' bodies, including their spinal columns, continue to grow through the teenage years. As a result, those hurt as children often face unique challenges in addition to the paralysis itself. For example, because their spines are not fully developed before puberty, trauma to the area can cause scoliosis (abnormal curvature of the spine), which sometimes requires bracing and/or surgery to correct. Although children with SCI are less likely than their adult counterparts to develop heterotopic ossification (abnormal growth of bone in soft tissues), they are more susceptible to hip dislocation and osteoporosis (weak, brittle bones) as they age.

Growing children and adolescents, with their increased bone metabolism, may develop a condition called immobilization hypercalcemia, in which blood levels of calcium are elevated. Boys in this age group with spinal cord injury are especially prone to this complication. Although some teenagers have no symptoms, others experience nausea and vomiting, malaise, and decreased appetite. These high levels of calcium can cause depression, so any young person with mood changes should have the calcium levels in his blood checked. Children and young adults with SCI should also be encouraged to eat a balanced diet rich in protein, iron, and vitamins to nourish their growing bodies.

Breathing and respiratory problems also differ depending on age; whereas paralyzed adults may be at elevated risk of pulmonary embolism, most children with SCI are not. But young people with cervical levels of injury are more susceptible to collapsed lungs and pneumonia, as well as to sleep apnea (when an individual temporarily stops breathing during sleep). Children are also at higher risk than adults for low blood pressure when changing from a sitting or lying position to an upright one (postural hypotension).

Incontinence and other bladder control problems also occur more often in injured people under the age of ten because their bladders have not yet reached full adult size (and, depending on the level of paralysis, may never do so). Because of the high likelihood of repeated infections, kidney and bladder stones are also more common in kids. Subsequently, doctors recommend intermittent catheterization, supervised or done by parents when necessary, instead of long-term (or indwelling) catheters. Children are usually able to begin learning how to do their own catheterization between the ages of five and eight, though adolescents may still need occasional reminders to carry out their bladder routine. Bowel and digestive challenges faced by kids are similar to those of injured adults, though enemas should be used more sparingly, since they may cause significant fluid imbalances and trigger autonomic dysreflexia (see Chapter 11) in young children.

Children are also still developing their cognitive and social skills, and these abilities (or inabilities) will affect how they come to handle their SCI. For example, kids who are born with spina bifida or are injured when they are very young will usually not be able to understand much of what makes them "different" from other kids. Children in general have a greatly simplified understanding of what is happening to them. Those who suddenly find themselves unable to walk or control their bodily functions at a time when they have not yet developed a strong self-image will need constant reassurance from their parents or other adults in their lives, in addition to help understanding their medical issues.

Because children are often less able than adults to articulate their feelings, they may have a more difficult time managing their anxieties, not only about doctors and medical procedures, but also about the future. While hospitalized, some children feel that they have been deserted by their parents or that they are being punished for some misbehavior. They don't yet have the emotional resources or experience to cope, and so some children with SCI may regress, refusing to do anything for themselves and demanding constant care from others—even when it's unnecessary. Being the center of attention often helps them manage their emotions.

Rehabilitation Issues

Since adults experience the majority of spinal cord injuries, most rehabilitation programs and equipment have been specifically designed to meet their needs rather than those of children and adolescents. In recent years, however, many rehabilitation centers have developed separate programs geared to their pediatric patients. There kids can live, interact, and participate in therapies alongside other kids with whom they share concerns and goals, as well as jokes and smiles. Rehabilitation regimens are tailored to meet the needs of different age groups, and emphasis is placed on preparing children psychologically for life with SCI, including their eventual return to school (helped, in some cases, by visits from educational specialists and tutors during inpatient rehab). The guiding principle of this vocational, educational, and social training for young patients is that people who are still growing and developing have excellent potential to regain their lives.

A child's home and school life before SCI also influences how he or she initially responds to injury and hospitalization. For example, kids who are already used to being away from their parents for extended periods of time, say, at boarding school or overnight summer camp, may have a slightly easier adjustment to hospital life than other kids, unless these previous separations have been unpleasant. On the other hand, for children who have experienced other stressful life-changing events, such as the illness or death of a close relative, hospitalization may bring back memories of those scary times. Some children may worry that their paralysis will push away those who love them, an ironic reaction since their relatives and loved ones are also often afraid of "losing" *them*. After years of caring for and protecting them, parents and guardians of young SCI patients are being forced to accept the fact that somebody else is now in charge of their children's health and well-being—at least during the initial hospitalization. (Family coping will be closely examined later in the chapter.)

Because a young child *is* dependent on his or her parents or other adult caregivers, grownups should learn as much as possible about their child's medical condition. Doctors, nurses, and other medical personnel can begin this process of education, which often goes a long way in aiding families as they attempt to provide comfort and emotional guidance to injured children while learning to cope themselves.

"The whole concept of a family-based approach is one of the biggest differences in treating kids; discussions about all the different aspects of SCI need to be done in a family context," explains Patrick Brennan, M.D., a pediatric physiatrist. "The most important thing is to listen first and see where a family is—what they've heard and what they've been told about prognosis, medical complications, and treatment. You know when they are ready to talk about the answers to tough questions when they start asking questions around them. You can talk directly to an adult with SCI, but you want to make sure parents are on the same page as you when you're dealing with their kids."

In talking to young patients about their condition, Brennan says that he often uses analogies and drawings to explain what's happening—referring to bowel and bladder issues, for instance, as "plumbing problems." In some cases, he says, even the youngest kids may be more ready than their parents to hear tough news. "Adults superimpose all their fears about what kids don't understand, but kids can ask tough questions. Answers need to be put in a form that meets their developmental stage. It's good, for instance, to ask parents how conversations have been handled when pets or relatives have died, or someone else has had a serious medical condition."

No matter how well children may adjust to being away from their parents, kids and teenagers in rehabilitation will inevitably experience many of the same fears and frustrations as older SCI patients—often without the maturity and sense of self to handle them. Lacking the grounding forces of a spouse, children, job, or their own home to focus on, they may easily become depressed or unsure of how they'll get by once they are discharged from the hospital. Many of them know nothing about spinal cord injury, and they may never even have talked to a person in a wheelchair. Because their lives are really just getting started, with educational and career dreams barely envisioned (if at all), they might have a harder time imagining a point of recovery. To them, only a moment before, it seemed that they had all the time in the world to have fun and figure out what they wanted to be; now, in an instant, many of these same options seem closed off. It's a scenario too frightening to be true; so perhaps, they hope, it's actually not real at all.

"When I was first hurt, I was joking around and didn't realize the seriousness of it," recalls Charlie, who was nineteen when a motorbike accident left him with C4-C5 tetraplegia. "I didn't feel anything, so I thought I was fine. My friends who were with me were acting the same way. I had no idea what tetraplegia was before I got hurt. When I heard someone "broke their neck" I figured they died. That's the way it is in the movies and video games. I couldn't feel anything below my neck, but I still thought I was getting some movement in my hands and arms. I figured I would be up and around in a day or two.

"Obviously this wasn't the case. Days turned into weeks, and it

seemed like I was in limbo with no sense of time at all. It was three or four weeks before I asked a doctor at one point, "Am I going to walk again?" and he said, "Probably not." Then I asked, "Am I going to get my arms back?" and he said, "You might get a little bit of shoulder shrugging."

Charlie's initial thought on hearing his diagnosis was "to push the doctor out the window." Rage, depression, and even suicidal thoughts among young people are not uncommon during hospitalization, and just as with adults, social contact with other paralyzed individuals undergoing rehabilitation can have a profoundly positive impact on them. Because children and teens with different levels of injury and at various stages of recovery participate in occupational and physical therapy sessions alongside other young patients in the therapy gym, the newer patients may learn better ways of coping and managing any feelings of sadness by observing and talking with those further along in their rehabilitation. The benefits may actually work *both* ways, as many young men and women with SCI have reported the tremendous sense of accomplishment and fulfillment they experience by going back and meeting with "rehab rookies" to provide them with support. In helping the newly injured, they are helping themselves as well.

Back Home: Rolling with the Changes

Challenges for Younger Children

While rehabilitation offers a chance to connect with other young people who are going through similar dramatic changes, paralyzed children and teens often face far greater challenges with their peers when they return to their "regular" life at home and school. Younger kids may find that old friends are hesitant to play with them, and that no longer having the freedom to ride a bike or maneuver the ins and outs of a playground puts them at a social disadvantage. The sight of a wheelchair may make some kids uncomfortable, especially if they have not been prepared for their classmate's return to school. Just as prearranged visits from oncology nurses can help educate the classmates of returning young cancer patients about the disease and what to expect, rehabilitation staff and parents can go a long way in combating prejudice and satisfying natural curiosity before a child with SCI reenters school.

Teachers can also help classes prepare for this transition by reading age-appropriate books on the subject. One of the most frequently recommended is *Rebecca Finds a New Way: How Kids Learn, Play, and Live with Spinal Cord Injuries and Illnesses* (published by the National Spinal Cord Injury Association in 1994). Written by Connie Panzarino, it tells the tale of seven-year-old Rebecca and her special friend Terry Terrific, a talking rabbit. One day Rebecca doesn't come home from school, and a worried Terry discovers that she has been in a car accident and is at the local hospital. Finding her unconscious in the intensive care unit, he waits until she awakens and learns she is paralyzed.

Throughout the rest of the story, Terry helps Rebecca adjust to her new life by talking with other kids in the rehab unit, returning with her to home and school, and eventually meeting new friends at a recreation program for children with disabilities. Serious issues like handling catheterization, using a respirator (as well as teaching others how to do so), and the disappointment of not being able to join friends in certain sports and activities are tackled in straightforward, easy-to-understand language. When Rebecca worries about whether her wheelchair will fit in her old room or if her catheter will work at home, for instance, she's voicing the same concerns of many SCI patients who might read her story.

Children in middle school can benefit from reading *How It Feels to Live with a Physical Disability*, a book that contains language and situations they can understand. Through extensive, poignant interviews, author Jill Kremetz introduces young readers to several children with different disabilities; among them is eleven-year-old Katherine, who was paralyzed in a plane crash when she was four. Katherine has faced not only the loss of her father, who was flying the plane and died in the crash, but also the challenge of rehabilitation, the return home, and reintegration into school, all at a very young age. Now, she says, she is "leading as normal a childhood as possible." During class she uses a standing board with a desktop attached so she can be at the same level as her schoolmates, and after school she enjoys swimming and playing tennis. Katherine states self-assuredly that "people who put me down are just putting themselves down, and I'm not going to let that stop me." She even shares a sure-fire way of handling big brothers that many younger siblings will applaud: "Whenever I get really mad at them, or their friends, I just run over their toes with my wheelchair. That usually keeps them from being mean to me for a while."

One issue on which paralyzed kids of all ages seem to agree is that they want teachers and classmates to treat them like everybody else. If a teacher pays special attention to them in class or grades them more easily, they feel uncomfortable. When friends struggle to talk with them, or avoid asking about their injury altogether as if it didn't happen, they feel bad then, too. Time and again, I've heard schoolkids with SCI say that they want to be accepted for who they are, injury and all. They don't mind educating others or explaining to their classmates and teachers what they can and can't do. (Younger kids can have a parent come in to help with this process.) As the ones living the experience, these newly injured children are best qualified to help "fill in the gaps" and bring things out in the open: in this way, they help eliminate their classmates' fear of the unknown as well as the stereotypes that others may project onto them. It's better, after all, to spread the word oneself than to have others talking about you.

A generation ago, before the Americans with Disabilities Act paved the way for many schools, playgrounds, and public places like movie theaters and shopping malls to become accessible, it was easy for children with SCI or other medical conditions that required wheelchairs to feel isolated from their peers. Today accessibility is far less of a factor, and with children in wheelchairs becoming increasingly visible in popular culture as well as in classrooms, it has become easier to "fit in" both physically and emotionally. Kids today grow up seeing wheelchair users on TV shows like "Sesame Street" and "Arthur," and they can buy dolls from "Mytwinn.com" and numerous other companies that come ready to go to school, work, the gym, or the big dance on two wheels rather than two legs.

In addition to helping children with SCI and other disabilities gain self-confidence, this changing landscape has also cut down on the most common experience faced by any kid who's different: teasing. "My experience with young children and their reaction to peers with disabilities or other situations requiring the use of a wheelchair or crutches is one of acceptance," says Elizabeth, a kindergarten teacher. "They are inquisitive and so curious to know what's 'wrong,' and want only to be reassured that the child in question is going to be OK. This generation of kids has been exposed to such a variety of abilities and disabilities in their young lives that it's truly amazing."

When it comes to talking about these differences, Elizabeth believes in being sensitive yet direct. "I firmly believe that presenting issues as honestly and openly as possible is the best way to go," she says. "I've found that if you speak to children at the appropriate developmental level, they are very open to differences of all kinds. In my classroom children are taught the definition of 'fair' when there is a child or children needing extra attention, time, or special 'equipment.' A friend in grad school once told me: 'Fair means everyone gets what they need.' Children are amazing creatures. They do not yet carry the adult 'junk' we've accumulated over the years that clouds our perceptions."

Congenital Paralysis

Julie and Paul had no idea what spina bifida was when their daughter Madison was delivered by emergency C-section, but they learned very quickly. She was in fetal distress, born with a malformation of the spinal cord, and surgery was needed to repair the abnormality. She returned home with her parents just ten days later, and each day since, the couple has worked to meet Madison's needs as a young girl with paraplegia as well as to give her (and their two other young children) as normal a life as possible. A few relatives living nearby have been very helpful, and they've depended a lot on the generosity of friends to help with babysitting and other necessities. "Although it was hard for us to ask for help in the beginning, we quickly learned to get good at it," says Paul. "You have to create a network of people you can depend on. Sometimes it's just setting people up to give you a monthly phone call and ask if you need anything. You learn both whom you can count on and to be specific about what you want."

Despite the challenges of being born paralyzed (her first five years included some ten operations), Madison is a happy seven-year-old who enjoys playing in the sandbox, blowing bubbles, and playing dress-up with her friends. Since she's the only child in a wheelchair at her suburban elementary school, however, her parents have had to stay on top of things. "Her school wasn't accessible between floors, so the only way to get from one floor to another was to go

outside and take a graded ramp in back of the school," explains
Julie. "That wouldn't work in winter, so we were able to get them to
put in a portable chair lift. The playground also wasn't accessible,
but we had a babysitter who raised $10,000 for the Spina Bifida As-
sociation running in a marathon, and we put those funds toward
the cost of a new playspace. The community was very caring; other
families in the school and the PTO also gave gifts to help cover the
$70,000 expense.

At school Madison enjoys "letting my friends push me in my
wheelchair at recess." Her parents have educated her classmates
about her condition, so she doesn't get too many odd stares or questions. If kids ask why she's in a wheelchair, she says simply, "My legs
can't move because of that spina bifida thing." (Sometimes, if they
don't feel comfortable asking her, classmates will question her parents.) Because teachers make a conscious effort not to treat her differently, her classmates generally don't think of her that way.

Nevertheless, her parents have devised guidelines for Madison's
playdates. "Inclusion and integration are a huge thing, but we still
run into some geographic restraints," says Julie. "It's hard for her
when the kids she's with all flow quickly into a new area where she
can't go. In addition to general accessibility issues, she has very low
muscle tone that makes it tougher for her to push her wheelchair
around. What we say to her friends is, 'If you're the last one to leave
a room and Madison is still there, make sure you tell an adult who
can carry her down to where you are.'" This goes for home, too,
where her brother and sister help her over thresholds and always remember to close the basement door so she can't accidentally fall
down the stairs.

"I like throwing balls into our trampoline and then making my
brother and sister get them," Madison says with a laugh. Her
brother isn't too keen on doing all the chasing, but when asked if he
ever wishes that his little sister could walk, he replies, "I don't think
so. Then she wouldn't be Madison."

Unlike children who must adjust to life with SCI at whatever age they are injured, kids who have spina bifida are paralyzed from birth. This congenital condition is a malformation of the spinal cord that actually starts when a baby is still inside the mother's womb. Because it usually occurs in the lower back, this birth defect will result in paralysis from the waist down—though many children still have *some* leg movement. Approximately 7 out of every 100,000 babies born in the United States have this complication, and more than 70,000 people in this country are currently living with it. Hispanic-Latino women are at greatest risk for having children with spina bifida, followed (in order) by whites, American Indians/Alaskan natives, blacks, and Asians/Pacific Islanders. This condition can be accompanied at times by another problem called hydrocephalus (also known as water on the brain), in which spinal fluid does not drain properly and excess pressure builds up in the infant's brain. Although spina bifida itself does not usually result in cognitive impairment, this can be the case when hydrocephalus is present.

As with SCI that results from accidents or other medical conditions, the degree of leg weakness that occurs in spina bifida can also vary from child to child. When the malformation occurs high in the spinal column, more muscles are affected and the child will most likely have to use a wheelchair. If the damage occurs lower down, fewer muscles are paralyzed and the child may learn to walk with crutches and braces. In some cases where the damage is at L5 or below, in fact, children may even be able to walk unaided, but like others with acquired SCI, they will also have compromised bowel and bladder control. Subsequently, they will need to follow specialized routines, either by themselves or with assistance, to prevent accidents.

Despite many similar challenges, children with paralysis since birth have one major advantage over those who become paralyzed—there is no period of adjustment or transition. They have never lived in a non-disabled body, so being disabled is a part of their identity. But while "different" is "normal" for them, it's not without its frustrations. Around age one, kids with SCI usually start to notice that their bodies are not the same as their peers'. This realization continues as they age; as six-year-olds on the playground, for instance, they may become discouraged as their friends start discovering the joys of the jungle gym.

At some point, usually around kindergarten, these children will notice the challenges that come with their differences, how their paralysis "disables" or limits them, and how others may perceive them as "less than normal." Just like those who become paralyzed as a result of an accident or an act of violence, they may become disappointed and even annoyed that they can't always do what their non-disabled peers can.

As Elizabeth the kindergarten teacher explains, how such kids view their disability and handle the discontent will depend in part on the reactions and responsiveness of others around them. For instance, the child who feels left out because of her inability to use the swings during recess will regard herself much differently than the boy who becomes the center of attention on the playground as classmates vie for rides with him on his wheelchair. Similarly, the paralyzed child whose parents show their despair as they watch her struggling to guide herself through town over bumps and curbs will have a much different experience of SCI than the boy whose family vocalizes their appreciation and respect for his alternate way of doing things and his resilience when facing challenges with creativity and motivation.

Many studies have shown that the most important influence on body image for *any* child is the attitude of parents and society, not his or her physical makeup. Kids need to be appreciated and loved by their parents; this solidifies their feelings of being complete and contributes to a healthy self-esteem. Yet parents of children with congenital SCI may experience emotional difficulties themselves that prevent them from giving their kids the support they need. Not unlike acquired paralysis, the condition also presents a major loss for parents, one that must be mourned and reconciled. But because the problem happened in utero (before birth), they may feel a different type of sadness and guilt. They have never had a chance to experience life with a "normal" child.

Some parents may wonder if the paralysis is the result of something the mother did, or didn't do, during pregnancy. Others may even see the condition as some kind of "divine punishment" for past transgressions. When a child feels that he or she is "normal" despite paralysis, these kinds of negative reactions by the parents may be quite confusing. Eventually, however, most parents are able to see the true potential of their disabled children, not just the limitations of SCI.

Challenges for Teenagers

"I'd struggle to get to class, things would be going along fine, and then all of a sudden I'd have a bowel accident," Danny remembers of his school days. "My day would be ruined, and I'd have to leave class to try to clean up. It stunk, and I'd be mortified. I had no warning. I'd be sitting in it and couldn't feel it. Urine accidents were another problem. To this day, twenty years later, I still have both problems. I can handle it now, but back then it was real tough."

Early childhood is often a time of uninhibited wonder and exploration, but by their teenage years many kids are starting to feel a need to "measure up" to their peers socially, physically, athletically, and academically. The pressure can be intense, and conformity of one type or another often gives relief and a sense of belonging to a stressed-out adolescent. At the same time a teen is trying to fit in, however, he or she may also be struggling to gain some measure of independence from parents, teachers, and other authority figures. Throw hormones, acne, and an uncertainty over "what to do with my life" into the mix, and you have an often fragile equilibrium. So while a spinal cord injury is disruptive no matter what a person's age, it can be particularly troublesome to those caught between being children and being grownups.

What are the biggest issues affecting the average teenager who becomes spinal cord injured? One problem is the sudden inability to drive—at least for the short term—a setback that for many kids means the end of "freedom" as they know it. Not being able to play mainstream sports or attend parties and school-related events that are held in inaccessible venues can also be devastating for teens. At school, depending on their level of injury, kids may be embarrassed by their need for an aide to help them get to and from classes, take notes, and even help them go to the bathroom or eat. If they are away at boarding school, camp, or college—the places where most teens relish their first true separation from parents—they may need an attendant just to get up each morning, shower and dress, and get out of their dorm room or cabin. Although a spinal cord injury will not hinder a young person's ability to develop fully into a mature man or woman, it can sometimes make any status-conscious teen feel like an outcast.

DATING DILEMMAS

"It's tough to talk to girls," admits Jeffrey, a seventeen-year-old who was injured two years ago. "I always wonder how they're looking at me. It's my fault that I think that way; I do it to myself. I make the wheelchair a kind of barrier, and I don't know how to get past it."

Dating and establishing relationships are among the greatest challenges faced by men and women with SCI (as addressed in

Chapter 5), and the same is true for teens. Those who had dated before their injury may be hesitant to "get out there again" because of a lack of confidence or the assumption that nobody will be interested in them. Teens who had little dating experience before paralysis will likely be more afraid than ever to take the step. Because physical appearance and the practice of "hooking up" are such significant components of the hormone-charged high school culture (and, increasingly, the middle school culture as well), it's impossible for newly injured kids *not* to think about it. Everywhere they look, it seems, kids are holding hands or making out while they sit in a corner. When a boy or girl *does* come over to talk, they wonder if the person is genuinely interested or just feels sorry for them. If they were in a steady relationship before they were hurt, teens with SCI may find themselves on the receiving end of a breakup because their boyfriend or girlfriend isn't comfortable being with somebody in a wheelchair or is overly concerned with what others will think.

The freedom and access a car can provide (including a convenient place to explore one's sexuality) are often not an option post-injury. Wheelchairs may not fit into the vehicles of friends, and having Mom or Dad in the cockpit of a specially modified van when you pick somebody up would likely rank with the most embarrassing of all high school situations. Well-intentioned friends and parents may suggest the logical solution of dating other paralyzed students, but most young people want the option of playing the entire field—not just the part of it that rolls. Fear of the awkward moments that lay ahead if they *do* get a date can also be a problem. Rather than deal with the uncomfortable act of asking someone for help at a restaurant or movie theater (not to mention the dilemma of going to the bathroom), paralyzed teens may opt to avoid the situation altogether.

For teenagers and kids of any age, learning to feel good about oneself again and turning this confidence into action is the key to getting back out there in all facets of life post-injury: school, extracurricular activities like art, music, or sports, a job, or even just hanging out with friends or family. When people see that someone is comfortable with his disability and confident about what he has to offer, they are much more likely to look beyond the chair and the awkward moments. Sometimes when teens come to accept their "new normal," that is, when they come to view themselves as individuals with spinal cord injury, they may, like paralyzed adults, be motivated to bond with others in the growing disabled network. In recent years numerous newsletters and websites (some listed in the Resources section at book's end) have appeared to give young people with SCI and other disabilities the chance to swap "war stories" and ideas on how to get by.

How Families React

Like the injured individuals themselves, most parents, siblings, extended family members, and friends often know little about paralysis until their loved one is affected. But because this group plays such an integral role in the lives of most children and adolescents, it is crucial that care during rehab and beyond be family-focused. Most people at this age are still living with their parents, so the more support that family members can provide to the injured person, the better the chances for a strong recovery. Whether they are aged five or ten or eighteen, the reassurance that children receive from their parents and close family members is as important to their well-being as the support of their caregivers—if not more so.

Parental Reactions

Dawn was a thirty-two-year-old single mother when doctors told her that her thirteen-year-old son, Justin, had suffered an injury to his C5-C6 spinal cord and would be paralyzed. As she recalls of those early days, "There was tons of disbelief on my part. He was fighting for his life on a ventilator, and all I cared about was whether he was going to survive. As they were talking to us, I couldn't absorb it. It was surreal. For three days straight, I was afraid if I went to bed I would wake up and he'd be gone. So I didn't go to sleep. After that, I started taking catnaps.

"Once they got him somewhat stable and he was in the ICU, they started asking me if I understood that he had a spinal cord injury. I was from a family of physicians, but this was outside all of our realms. I didn't know what was affected in such cases, or all the bowel and bladder issues involved. I was horrified when I heard about cathing for the first time. The severity of it still had not sunk in, and I wasn't ready to accept that this was a forever thing." Getting to meet and talk with parents of other SCI patients during rehab was helpful, but Dawn still wondered if she would be able to handle the challenges ahead. Nor could she understand how her son could be so upbeat in such a seemingly desperate situation.

"Sometimes I was so angry at the beginning, and I wondered why he wasn't more upset himself," she says. "I wanted to shake him to get him to go through the whole grieving process with me. All he would do is say, 'Mom, at least I'm still here.' Once I came to accept the seriousness of the situation, what was important for me was to make sure that whatever steps we took helped him become more independent, because it's just the two of us. Often the steps you take wind up making the people you're trying to help more dependent, and I didn't want that to happen to Justin."

All parents have dreams for their children: to see them grow up healthy, happy, and strong; excel in school, sports, and other activities; enjoy professional success in a rewarding career; and, possibly, fall in love and have their own kids. In a split second, a spinal cord injury seems to end all these hopes and aspirations. As a parent looks down at a child hooked up to tubes in the intensive care unit and is told that this beloved son or daughter may never walk again, it feels as if everything is lost. In the case of life-threatening injuries, survival is usually the primary concern early on. Those days during which the outcome is uncertain are harrowing, as any parent whose child is hurt feels immense despair and helplessness at not being able to protect him or her from such pain and danger. Once the patient has stabilized, however, the focus shifts to how the child is going to live as an individual with paraplegia or tetraplegia—and it is here that the unique and very challenging role that parents play in recovery comes into full force.

GETTING THROUGH GRIEF, GUILT, AND ANGER

Parents spend years mending bumps and bruises both physical and mental, tending to every tear and nightmare. But SCI is something that Mom and Dad *cannot* fix—something that threatens to disrupt much of what they have done to help guide their children along the best and safest path possible. Feelings of grief and guilt about their powerlessness to improve the situation or keep it from happening in the first place are only natural, and often take some time and effort to work through. Accordingly, parents may experience intense sorrow, not just for their child, but also for their own loss. Others may try to repress their feelings of anger toward the newly paralyzed out of a sense that such a reaction is unacceptable. This bottled-up anger, however, can further damage parental self-esteem and expend emotional energy.

No matter the reactions, it is important that parents do work through them so that their feelings don't hinder the rehabilitation process. Only when emotional pain is experienced can it be conquered. Once parents confront their emotions they can look forward and deal with life's challenges, learning to accept what cannot be changed and reconciling with their new reality. The same is true, of course, for grandparents, uncles and aunts, and other family caregivers who are raising or helping to raise children with SCI.

Another type of unspoken guilt or angst may develop as parents question whether they are even able to handle the challenge of caring for a paralyzed child. Especially if their son or daughter is completely dependent, they may, at brief moments, wish for some relief from this responsibility. As instantly as these thoughts enter their heads, in most cases, the love they have for their child tends to overpower the negativity, but not before a big dose of guilt enters as well. It's important for parents to realize that such reactions are completely natural and nothing to be ashamed of. Just because they sometimes feel overwhelmed by the responsibility does not mean that they love their child any less; it just means that they're human.

"No one wants to be a caregiver forever, but you feel like that's your role sometimes," says Julie, mother of young Madison, who has spina bifida. "In some cases you're faced with the prospect of permanent loss earlier than most people, and some folks don't want to learn too much about us and our struggles. It touches their own vulnerabilities." Good friends, however, can often be a big help to parents in getting through the days. "Some people have a knack for just knowing, and will drop off a meal or do something else without asking," she says. "That's the best kind of help, when somebody just seems to read your mind."

Although the natural tendency of parents is to protect their children from harm, too much coddling can have detrimental effects in the long run. This overprotection is sometimes an offshoot of guilt; parents who feel responsible for not being able to prevent their son's or daughter's injury might try to do everything possible for the child from that point onward. But just as adults with SCI need to move ahead and regain their independence after an initial adjustment period, younger individuals facing these circumstances should do the same. Even though the family will be there for support, encouragement, and help, and the knowledge of their presence is a source of comfort for paralyzed people of *all* ages, injured children need to start doing things for themselves, like coming to the table for meals or cleaning their rooms, as soon as they can. Young kids as well as teenagers need structure and discipline in order to thrive, and parents should not shirk in providing either just because their son or daughter is in a wheelchair.

Continuing to bathe and serve meals in bed to an injured child who is functioning at an independent level, for instance, does no good for either party. The child doesn't learn how to fend for him- or herself; nor are the parents helping him or her to reach this point. Just as parents may appropriately encourage an able-bodied son or daughter to excel in school, on the athletic field, or in the community, so, too, should they assist that same youngster with these or other, redefined goals *after* injury. Although a paralyzed individual may always require some degree of help, the key for parents is to not let their desire to offer this assistance supersede their role as the major guiding force in their children's development.

It is better for parents to do everything possible to push their son or daughter toward more independence in each facet of their lives—a move that is definitely in the best interests of the injured child. Helping their kids to build self-esteem will enable them to establish realistic academic, social, and professional goals. By becoming advocates for disability at school and in the community, parents can ensure that accessibility is the norm and that teachers and other leaders are sensitive to their children's needs. Just as most adults with SCI find they can adapt to their injuries and go on to lead meaningful lives filled with personal and professional successes, parents will eventually realize that their children can accomplish a great deal—and that they can help them get there.

FOCUSING ON THE WHOLE FAMILY

In caring for their disabled child, parents must also consider his or her siblings. If they have other young sons or daughters living at home, they need to focus as much attention on them as on the child in the wheelchair (if not as much actual assistance). Siblings often feel slighted by all the extra concern being given to the injured child. Parents in this situation can help the entire family by letting *every* child know that he or she is important, by making sure to give each special time and reinstating as many familiar and fun routines into the household as possible—even something as simple as a trip to the park or ice cream store. In addition to helping brothers and sisters feel better, this practice will help alleviate some of the injured child's guilt about "ruining everything" because of his or her paralysis.

This isn't to say that the household will not face major changes, however. The family may need to move to a more accessible home or even a different community so the paralyzed child can be closer to a particular school or hospital. Finances may become tight as insurance runs out or parents are faced with taking out a second mortgage on their home to help pay for personal care attendants, equipment, and other needs. If the daily responsibilities of raising a paralyzed child grow particularly demanding, one parent may feel pressure to quit his or her job and stay at home (if they don't already). In families where there is only one parent, or divorced parents who both have homes in which the child spends time—perhaps even as a stepchild or stepsibling—different logistical and emotional challenges may emerge. These will affect how the family functions as one, but with honesty, commitment, and a lot of effort, parents can work through them.

Sibling Reactions

Because they were only a year apart in age, Paula and Betsy had always been more like best friends than sisters. Although at seventeen Paula was the older one, they hung out with the same friends and in some cases even dated a few of the same boys. When a car accident left Paula with tetraplegia, however, the dynamics of their relationship changed considerably. Suddenly, rather than remaining inseparable buddies, they experienced a change in their bond as the younger sibling now took on the "big sister" role. Although they still spent a lot of time together, it was mostly when Betsy helped Paula shower, dress, and get out the door each day. At the mall, though both girls were still approached by boys, Betsy was the one with whom they flirted. And though Paula did remain popular with her classmates, Betsy often went out alone on the weekends because many of the parties they got invited to were held in inaccessible homes.

It was not easy for Paula to watch her able-bodied sister continue to do all the things they used to do together as a pair. And even though she loved Betsy and appreciated the help she gave her, Paula was ashamed to admit that she felt a little angry and jealous as well. Betsy, in turn, was happy to help her sister, but she hated to admit that she was a bit stressed because of all the time her assistance took away from daily homework and extracurricular activities. Even when she did get away for a social break at someone's house, Betsy felt guilty if the house was not accessible and Paula was left out. Most of all, both worried if the close relationship they had always shared could survive all the changes.

Next to parents, the individuals most affected by a young person's spinal cord injury are his or her siblings. Having already formed their bonds before SCI, paralyzed children and their brothers and sisters often must reevaluate their relationships within the context of the new situation. The jealousy and rivalry that can often be found in even the healthiest of young sibling bonds can reemerge or intensify following a catastrophic event of this type, as can resentment if able-bodied children feel that their parents are paying less attention to them and more to their injured brother or sister. This bitterness can be compounded if the sibling, like Betsy, is also being asked to provide some or much of the care required by the paralyzed child. If a sibling can be upfront about how much he or she truly wants (or is able) to help, some of the tension may decrease before the situation gets out of control and a wedge forms between brothers and/or sisters.

Parents can assist in the transition from the start by having their able-bodied children take part in planning how the family will adapt to the paralyzed sibling's return home from the hospital or rehab center. This may include housing modifications (such as moving the returning child to a first-floor bedroom, as well as helping to decorate it), figuring out which chores he or she can still do, and which need to be given to others, and taking a trip to the market to stock up on his or her favorite foods. Assuming that the returnee will probably dominate much of the parents' time at first, moms and dads might want to participate in special activities with their other kids ahead of time—even if it's only a movie or a basketball game in the driveway. The goal in all cases is to make the return home a positive and natural step for the family, and to alleviate some of the anxiety that siblings—and everybody in the household—may be feeling. Even if a family camping trip or a week at the beach needs to be temporarily postponed, *all* the kids in the house should be made to feel special and taken care of during this challenging period.

Once the injured child is back in the home, it is best that brothers and sisters leave such tasks as bathing and bowel and bladder care to others and *not* become personal care attendants for their siblings. This is the same advice I often give to partners of individuals with SCI (see Chapter 7). Occasionally lending a helping hand is fine, but by waiting on a brother or sister with drinks, books, and TV remotes, siblings can actually do more harm than good. Constantly providing assistance of this kind may send the message to the newly injured child that she doesn't have to worry about taking care of herself, which can be a detriment to her adjustment. It can also lead to resentment that simmers below the surface and has the potential to seriously disrupt the household's equilibrium.

"Sometimes if I'm playing catch with my dad, Madison will say she wants a turn," eight-year-old Paul Jr. says of his younger sister. "So she'll throw it to my dad, and he'll throw it to me. Danielle, our little sister, is able to stand on the back of Madison's wheelchair and watch." Helping deflect some of the questions at school is also a great job for big brothers or sisters. "A kid in Madison's class sometimes asks me questions, but mostly it's people who come to our house and ask why she can't walk," explains Paul Jr. "At school they know she's in a wheelchair, but they think she goes home and gets up out of it."

Children with SCI often benefit from having able-bodied siblings at home or school with whom they can discuss their concerns about adjusting to life in a wheelchair. During adolescence an injured child may rebel against the restrictions of his condition and direct this anger toward his parents. Brothers and sisters can play a crucial role in helping a paralyzed teen through these challenging years by serving as unconditional advocates and sounding boards. As these siblings grow into adults, the likelihood is good that this familial bond will continue as an especially strong and satisfying one for all involved.

In the end, many people can help a paralyzed child as he or she begins to reintegrate into the world: family, friends, caregivers, teachers, and others. The hope is that each child faced with this challenge can be accepted back with the understanding and encouragement necessary to take the scary first steps. Nobody, however, can make the process work if the injured person doesn't want it for him- or herself. The road back can be a tough one, especially given all the bumps along the way that most young people encounter. Nonetheless, the potential benefits of a satisfying life now and into adulthood make it a trip worth taking. Those who have already made much of the journey can attest to this fact; as Katherine, the eleven-year-old girl with paraplegia interviewed for Jill Krementz's book, states, "If someone asked me to describe myself, I would say I'm a person who can't walk but who can do everything else."

Medical Complications of SCI: Do's and Don'ts

Bobby, a construction worker injured in a job-related fall, actively participated in rehab for C8 tetraplegia and returned home after three months. Early the next spring he went to his first baseball game in a wheelchair, accompanied by his teenage son. "We had such a great time that we stayed until the last pitch, even though the Red Sox were way ahead and the heat was terrible," he recalls. "But then, just as we were getting up to leave, I felt a headache coming on. By the time we reached the main gate, the pounding was getting worse and I started feeling anxious."

Bobby's son noticed his dad's flushed face and excessive sweating and ran to the first aid booth to call for an ambulance. In the emergency room, Bobby's blood pressure was checked. With a reading of 190/100 (normal for him was 90/60), the nurse knew exactly what was going on: autonomic dysreflexia. She sat him up immediately, loosened his belt, and asked when he had last emptied his bladder. "It was only then," explains Bobby, "that I realized I had been having so much fun at the game that I hadn't catheterized myself in eight hours, even though I drank two large bottled waters and a jumbo lemonade."

This was all the nurse needed to hear; she quickly "cathed" Bobby, removing 900 milliliters of urine. Almost instantly, his pain subsided and his blood pressure normalized. Once he was feeling better, the nurse went upstairs to the hospital's rehab unit and returned with a card for Bobby to keep in his wallet. Emblazoned with

the heading "Medical Alert for Autonomic Dysreflexia," it listed the
warning signs for this serious medical complication faced by many
paralyzed individuals, along with how to manage it. Bobby prom-
ised to commit the card to memory, as well as to watch the clock
more carefully when it came to his bowel and bladder care—even at
the ballpark.

Having a spinal cord injury means more than just not being
able to move your arms or legs. Because the spinal cord affects
many significant bodily functions, it is important for individuals
and their families to be aware of the possible medical complications that can occur after paralysis. With proper knowledge and
initiative, however, people can learn to recognize the warning
signs of the various conditions detailed in the pages that follow,
as well as to take the appropriate preventative measures. Furthermore, knowing how to get the necessary treatment is crucial
if any one of these complications does arise.

Types of Complications

Autonomic Dysreflexia (AD)

Also called autonomic hyperreflexia, or "going hyper," autonomic
dysreflexia (AD) is one of the few potential medical emergencies
that a person with SCI must be aware of. This condition can
cause extremely high blood pressure and thereby increase the
risk for stroke, seizures, and even death. The condition usually
affects only those individuals with paralysis at or above the sixth
thoracic level (T6), though it has also been reported on rare occasions in injuries as low as T8. Although many people will first
experience a dysreflexic episode during their inpatient rehabilitation stay, where it can be managed by the nurses and doctors,
others, like Bobby, may have their first such experience away

from the hospital, after discharge. Some may never encounter this condition at all, however, even if their level of paralysis puts them at risk. Nonetheless, since it can happen anytime after a spinal cord injury (or at least, once a person's muscle reflexes return), everyone who is at risk—and their families— must know how to recognize, treat, and prevent this potentially life-threatening event.

Autonomic dysreflexia occurs when the body experiences something that before SCI would have caused pain or discomfort, like a full bladder or skin burn, but now goes unnoticed because of decreased sensation. When this kind of "noxious" event happens to an able-bodied person, messages are sent to the brain alerting the individual of pain and the need to remedy it. A spinal cord injury prevents this communication, however. As a result (perhaps to provide some sort of warning), the body reacts with excessive nervous system activity—a "hyper" reflex—that raises blood pressure and causes blood vessels below the level of injury to tighten.

Above the injury, vessels stay open to counteract the elevated blood pressure, and the blotchy, red face that results is a typical sign that someone is experiencing autonomic dysreflexia. Other common symptoms include a severe pounding headache, nausea, nasal congestion, anxiety, or irritability. Some people describe blurred or spotty vision (resulting from elevated blood pressure), and those witnessing the episode may notice that the person is sweating above the level of injury and has cold, clammy skin below it. In response to the high blood pressure, the heart rate frequently slows as well.

It is crucial for those at risk and their loved ones to recognize the signs of autonomic dysreflexia quickly and respond appropriately. AD has often been mistaken for an isolated headache or even a head cold, but when the person has the described level of paralysis, as well as an elevation in blood pressure, the diagnosis is definitely AD. First, the person should sit up; elevation of the trunk relative to the legs causes the blood pressure to drop as blood pools in the lower limbs. Second, the cause of the episode (examples to follow) must be determined and removed. Until this inciting factor is alleviated, the symptoms will continue—and may even worsen.

The most common source of dysreflexia is a full and over-distended bladder. While failure to catheterize the bladder is a common trigger, AD can also occur when an indwelling catheter becomes clogged, or the tubing kinked, preventing urine from flowing. In this case, the treatment is simple: sit up and empty the bladder or clear the blockage. Since catheterization alone has the potential to cause dysreflexia (by stimulating the nervous system), anyone with AD who needs to use a catheter should put anesthetic jelly on it to decrease any excess sensory input and avoid aggravating the problem.

Other possible irritants that can lead to autonomic dysreflexia include urinary tract infections; constipation; pressure sores; tight-fitting clothing; ingrown toenails; and burns (including sunburns). If a person develops AD, always consider the most common and obvious causes first. For example, after ensuring that the bowel and bladder are empty, examine the skin for any signs of pressure, cuts, or bruises, and then make sure that clothing is not too tight. Inspect fingers and toes for ingrown nails as well. If you cannot find the cause, and if the elevated blood pressure persists, seek medical attention as soon as possible. Sometimes bladder, kidney, or gallstones; stomach ulcers; or even severe menstrual cramps can lead to autonomic dysreflexia. Until the source can be identified, medication may be used to lower the blood pressure.

Overall, prevention is the best way to manage AD. Most causes of dysreflexia (but not all) can be avoided by practicing good self-care. The bladder, for example, should not be allowed to become too full. Catheterization should be done on a regular schedule, and indwelling catheters should be checked during the day to make sure they are draining adequately. Bowel programs also must be followed carefully to prevent constipation. In addition, frequent skin checks and pressure relief are essential to prevent skin breakdown, or pressure sores.

Another important step to AD prevention and health maintenance after SCI is establishing and maintaining a relationship with a physician who is knowledgeable about spinal cord injury and its possible complications. Additionally, people at risk for dysreflexia (that is, those with injuries at T6 or above) should carry a card in their wallet like the one given to Bobby describing the condition, its causes, and proper treatment methods so as to alert medical professionals and/or hospitals lacking adequate experience with AD.

Spasticity

Stacey was a thirty-year-old woman with T5 paraplegia as a result of a car accident. During rehab, she learned that daily range-of-motion exercises were an excellent way to keep her arms and legs limber as she prepared to, and then resumed, her active life as the mother of two elementary-age children. Practicing her stretching program diligently, she returned home independently in a wheelchair and was soon back helping with the neighborhood carpool in an SUV equipped with hand controls. "Several months later, I noticed my legs getting stiffer, and it was harder to get in and out of bed or transfer to the car," she recalled. "I kept doing my stretching exercises, but they didn't seem to help anymore. My doctor prescribed a medication called baclofen, but the problem only got worse. My leg spasms started keeping me up at night, and one time I almost fell out of my wheelchair. I called my doctor back, and he increased the dose, but all that did was make me sleepy all the time. It got to the point where I didn't even feel safe driving."

Then, at a support group meeting for mothers with disability,

Stacey heard about another treatment option: a baclofen pump. In-
stead of taking her medication by mouth, she could now have it de-
livered directly to her spinal cord via this round, surgically implanted
device, and in such small doses that her energy level would not be
affected. Encouraged by the success that others had experienced,
Stacey decided the operation to implant the pump was just what
she needed—and made an appointment with a neurosurgeon to dis-
cuss it further.

Although people with SCI have limited ability to *voluntarily*
move their arms and/or legs, some develop problems with too
much *involuntary* muscle movement. This exaggerated activity
is called spasticity (or hypertonicity) and varies for each individual. (In contrast, people with damage to the spinal cord at
the lower lumbar or sacral area—that is, the *cauda equina,* discussed in Chapter 1—have the opposite problem: their legs
will usually be loose or flaccid.) People with spasticity complain
that their muscles are tight or rigid and difficult to move owing to increased muscle tone, and they may also be bothered
by random and spontaneous movements of their limbs, called
spasms.

Spasticity occurs after paralysis because of the altered communication between the brain and the muscles that are involved
below the level of the injury. Normally, for a muscle to move, the
brain transmits a message to the part of the spinal cord that controls the muscle, and a contraction occurs. Next the muscle
sends feedback to the brain regarding how much it has moved,
whether it is painful, and so on. The brain may then send inhibi-
tory chemicals to the muscles to modulate their activity and improve motor control.

With a spinal cord injury, however, the brain won't receive this
kind of feedback information about excessive muscle movements,
and spasticity subsequently results—like a reflex from the spinal

cord. This same sort of reaction results when a person touches a hot stove; the immediate movement of his or her hand away from the heat occurs without any processing by the brain. In this reflex reaction, just as the fingers touch the burner, the spinal cord receives "noxious" sensory information and immediately causes the hand and arm muscles to move. The brain is not involved.

Spasticity can cause either a single, brief muscle contraction or more prolonged and repetitive muscle movements. The condition can cause hips and knees to bend (flexor spasms), or the knees or torso to forcefully straighten (extensor spasms). Unfortunately, spasms can be not only a nuisance but also a source of severe pain that limits a person's function. For example, spasticity in the trunk or legs can interfere with transferring out of bed or walking because of the decreased flexibility. Some increased tone in the fingers can leave hands in a clenched-fist position, causing stiffness and making it difficult to keep them clean as fingers become tight. Other times, involuntary spasms are just bothersome, like a foot that keeps moving and wakes a person at night. Spasms that go untreated may lead to skin irritation and pressure sores from the constant friction between the skin and clothing or bed sheets. At the extreme, contractures can occur, whereby the soft tissues surrounding muscles and joints become so tight that the joint can no longer be moved.

For some people, spasticity can actually be a *good* thing. Because it makes them contract, this process helps muscles maintain their bulk and keep bones strong. Some specialists believe that it may even prevent blood clots by keeping muscles moving. Moreover, some individuals actually use their spasticity to maintain their trunk position during transfers from bed to wheelchair and the like, or to keep their legs stiff and supportive for walking with braces. Under the right circumstances, spasticity of the bladder muscles can even help a person empty his or her bladder. In other cases, however, an increase in spasticity can indicate the presence of a urinary tract infection, kidney stones, ingrown toenails, or the initial stages of a pressure sore. In this way, spasticity can serve as a "warning system" for serious health problems that might otherwise go unrecognized. It may even be a precursor to an episode of autonomic dysreflexia.

When attempting to prevent spasticity, the best approach is to eliminate any stimulus that might exacerbate it, like bladder infections or skin problems. Most people who have only mild spasticity find that regular stretching and range-of-motion exercises are enough to keep their muscles loose. Some may also use resting splints on their arms and/or legs to keep their hands and feet in proper position and prevent discomfort. Since stress can worsen increased tone, general relaxation methods like breathing exercises and meditation have been helpful in moderating spasms. Yoga can also be beneficial for individuals with SCI, as it emphasizes mind-body wellness and helps with overall relaxation. The different asanas, or postures used in yoga, in fact, can easily be modified for those seated in a wheelchair. Warm water baths or pools and massage can also bring good results. In addition, since caffeine can worsen spasms, tapering off caffeinated beverages and chocolate could improve muscle tone.

If spasticity begins to interfere with mobility and self-care and cannot be adequately managed with stretching and positioning alone, medications may be necessary. Antispasticity drugs are taken by mouth and work by relaxing tight muscles directly or through the spinal cord or brain. Unfortunately, some of these agents—which include baclofen (lioresal), tizanidine, and diazepam—may have side effects such as drowsiness, dizziness, or even liver damage. In most cases, when I treat spasticity, I try one medication at a time, and then, depending on the results, either add or substitute a second one to obtain the best patient response with the fewest complications.

When a specific body part, rather than the entire body, is affected by spasticity, antispasticity agents can be directly injected into the involved muscle or nerve. Alcohol and phenol have been used in this way for many years, for instance, as a means to straighten an arm bent at the elbow or to unclench fingers closed in a fist. These "blocks," also known as neurolysis, are usually performed by a neurologist or a physiatrist in the office setting. They are permanent and occasionally may cause some unwanted weakness as well as uncomfortable burning sensations. Now that botulinum toxin is commercially available for injection, is easier to administer than traditional blocks, and has fewer side effects, it is frequently the agent of choice to treat localized spasticity affecting a particular muscle. The response takes two to three days for full effect, and repeat injections are necessary every three months.

For those with generalized spasticity who derive minimal help from or cannot tolerate oral medications because of the side effects, the baclofen pump offers another option. For this technique a titanium reservoir, the size of a hockey puck, is surgically implanted beneath the skin in the lower abdomen and connected to a catheter that dispenses liquid baclofen directly into the spinal canal at a controlled rate and frequency. Because only 1/100th of the typical dose of baclofen is necessary, side effects from the drug are minimal and the potential to control spasticity greater. Every month or two the doctor refills the pump by injecting baclofen directly into the reservoir; the pump itself must be replaced every four to five years. Because the pump has been so successful, many surgical procedures previously used to manage spasticity have been almost completely abandoned. These include tenotomies, in which tendons are cut, or the dorsal rhizotomy, whereby nerve branches from the spinal cord are destroyed to interrupt the spastic reflex. Although spasticity is still difficult to eliminate completely, it has definitely become more manageable.

Deep Venous Thrombosis (DVT) and Pulmonary Embolism (PE)

Walking helps keep blood flowing in the body because contracting leg muscles act like pumps. Subsequently, a person who uses a wheelchair will have reduced "pumping ability" and, therefore, less effective circulation. When blood is stagnant and pools in the lower extremities, it may solidify and form a clot in a vein. This condition, known as deep venous thrombosis (DVT), obstructs blood flow and may result in increased swelling and/or leg pain. In the worst-case scenario, the clot can break free and travel up the body into the lungs, a life-threatening situation called pulmonary embolism.

The most common warning signs of DVT are increased calf tenderness, swelling, and/or warmth. The problem is that many other things can cause these same symptoms, including infection, heterotopic ossification (to be discussed next), muscle strain, or fracture, making this condition quite difficult to diagnose. Moreover, a clot can occur without any definitive signs, sometimes just a low-grade fever around 100 degrees. With a pulmonary embolism (PE), a sudden rapid heartbeat, shortness of breath, chest tightness (especially when taking in a deep breath), or a sudden fever may occur. If a person with paralysis develops these symptoms (particularly in the context of reduced activity, like bedrest during an illness), urgent medical attention is required.

Prevention is once again the key. Because of the difficulty detecting a DVT or a PE, as well as their potential seriousness, pneumatic compression stockings or elastic bandages wrapped around the legs are usually recommended during periods of inactivity or bedrest. Range-of-motion exercises will also help keep blood circulating throughout the extremities, as will the spontaneous muscle spasms mentioned previously. When a person is on bedrest or hospitalized, a medication called heparin, which is injected into the stomach several times a day, is used to thin blood and prevent clots. When a clot does occur, higher doses of a special type of heparin may be given twice daily; another option is using an oral blood thinner called warfarin for several months.

Heterotopic Ossification (HO)

Ted Purcell was a twenty-year-old college student who excelled at many sports until a wipeout during a particularly challenging ski jump left him with low tetraplegia. Although he was motivated to get back to school and the slopes as soon as possible, he was sidetracked by a problem during rehabilitation. Painful bone deposits formed in his hip joints, and the resulting restrictions in flexibility left him unable to do many of the independent tasks such as dressing that a person with his level of injury normally could. Because the bones were still growing, doctors felt it best to wait before performing surgery. "Eventually they went in with a hammer and chisel and whacked them out," Ted recalls. "Then I had two weeks of radiation so the deposits wouldn't grow back. I had to take this awful medicine, and, knock on wood, they've never come back. They said I might develop pretty weak hip joints as a result, but twenty years later that hasn't happened yet."

This condition, called heterotopic ossification (HO), can afflict people with spinal cord injuries and other disabilities like strokes and brain injuries. Bits of bone grow within the body's soft tissues, often near a joint, in areas where there is usually no bone. In general, no one knows why this occurs, or why it happens to some people with SCI but not others. One thing is clear: heterotopic ossification arises only in joint areas *below* the level of injury. In people with paraplegia, for example, only the hips, thighs, and knee areas can be affected, while those with tetraplegia may develop this "extra" bone near their elbows as well.

The usual signs of heterotopic ossification are swelling, redness, warmth, and/or pain around the involved joint. If these symptoms appear, it is important to exclude the presence of other serious conditions, including deep venous thrombosis, a fracture, infection, or more rarely, a tumor. The most serious potential complication of HO is the reduced joint movement that can occur when a significant amount of bone grows. Depending on the location of this extra bone, limitations in joint mobility may make wheelchair seating/positioning and self-care tasks more challenging.

Various tests are available to detect and monitor the growth of this condition. One blood test measures levels of alkaline phosphotase, a blood chemical that increases when the heterotopic ossification is actively growing, then drops back to normal when it stops developing. This lab test serves as a helpful marker of the bones' activity, though other conditions (including fractures) can also cause an elevation in alkaline phosphotase. Until about four to ten weeks after the process has begun, X-rays will not show the presence of heterotopic ossification, nor can they indicate how long it has been there. Bone scans, which are performed using a special camera that detects labeled radioactive material injected into the bloodstream, can detect HO about four weeks earlier than X-rays—and can also determine if the bone is mature (actively growing) or not.

Once heterotopic ossification is diagnosed, the best way to manage it is to keep the joints moving and prevent any restrictions by doing regular gentle, passive, range-of-motion exercises. Some physicians will prescribe anti-inflammatory medications for HO, since inflammation is thought to trigger this abnormal bone growth. The only medication considered to be of any use for the condition, however, is etidronate. This drug may stop the existing heterotopic ossification from growing further and prevent any new areas from forming, but it does not alter the bone that already exists. If joint mobility does become limited by the presence of HO and problems with mobility or self-care result, surgery is an option to remove, or at least reduce, the extra bone. Surgeons will operate only if the bone is determined to be mature and no longer actively growing as seen on a bone scan. This may take several months to a year. But if the individual's range of motion and fundamental abilities are *not* affected, this extra bone is usually just treated conservatively and left alone.

Pressure Sores

Skin, muscle, and bone need a constant supply of blood and oxygen to stay healthy. Yet when a person remains in the same position for an extended time, as in a wheelchair, pressure increases to certain body parts such as the buttocks and the thighs. This, in turn, *decreases* circulation to these areas. When this reduced blood flow occurs in people who do not have a spinal cord injury, they experience an uncomfortable sensation in the affected area, causing them to shift their position. Blood flow is subsequently restored, and the discomfort alleviated. (This commonly occurs, for example, during movies or religious services, when attendees stay in one position for extended periods of time.) In contrast, individuals with paralysis have diminished sensation and do not receive these same pain messages from the nerve endings. As a result, they may remain in the same position without shifting their body weight, thereby cutting off the essential nutrients needed by skin and soft tissue. If blood flow is reduced for long enough, cells will die and skin will begin to break down.

Pressure sores vary in severity, from a simple area of redness on the skin that lasts five or more minutes after pressure is relieved (known as a stage one ulcer), to deeper areas that extend to the muscle and/or bone (stage three or four ulcers). If pressure sores go unnoticed and untreated, they can eventually result in infection. Sometimes people have had to have limbs amputated when soft tissue infections become so extensive that they cannot be treated any other way.

FIGHTING BACK

Unfortunately, the majority of people with SCI develop pressure sores at some point during their lifetimes. Elevated pressure is not the only factor that contributes to this development; friction, moisture, malnutrition, smoking, and advanced age can also increase a person's risk. Vigilant skin care is the best way to avoid this complication, since most skin breakdown is preventable. On the first day of rehabilitation, the treatment team and I instruct patients and their families and/or caregivers to inspect their skin at least twice daily, looking for the early signs of prolonged pressure like redness or skin tears. I usually recommend that these skin checks be done right after awakening in the morning and once before bed, with particular attention to bony body parts (like the tailbone, hips, and heels), which are at high risk for skin breakdown (see Figure 10). For tough-to-see areas, occupational therapists often give people long-handled flexible mirrors in aid in skin inspection. (If a person has limited grip, straps are added to the mirror to assist in use.)

Additionally, equipment such as braces and wheelchair cushions need to be closely monitored and maintained, since skin problems can occur if they break or don't fit correctly. Clothing must also be just the right size, since a tight waistband may add

Pressure Points

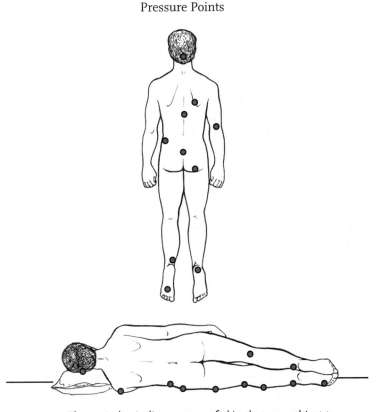

FIGURE 10.   These circles indicate areas of skin that are subject to high pressure—and skin breakdown—when an individual lies on his back (top diagram) or on his side (bottom) for long periods of time. People with decreased sensation should inspect such areas as part of their daily health-maintenance routine.

unnecessary pressure to the skin and hinder circulation. On the other hand, clothing that is *too* loose may cause wrinkles that can also press against the skin and cause breakdown.

In meeting with patients, I constantly reinforce the importance of good positioning and frequent pressure relief in their day-to-day lives. Pressure relief for people with SCI basically means repositioning themselves frequently during the day. This helps to maintain blood flow to tissue, which, in turn, prevents skin breakdown and improves tissue healing if pressure ulcers should occur. For those who use a wheelchair, the buttocks are at particularly high risk for pressure sores, as discussed earlier. I recommend shifting weight in one's chair for thirty seconds every fifteen minutes. This can be done independently or with assistance, depending on the person's upper-body strength.

In an anterior weight shift, the person bends forward at the waist, bringing his head between his thighs and knees. To reduce pressure on the posterior thighs, the person leans to one side in a wheelchair (after removing an armrest), and then to the other. People who have adequate arm strength can perform the "wheelchair push-up": with their hands on armrests, they extend their elbows and lift their buttocks off the cushion, thereby restoring circulation. Some of my patients wear watches with alarms that go off every fifteen minutes to remind them to do their pressure relief.

For those with tetraplegia who cannot do their own pressure relief, electric weight-shifting wheelchair systems are available. The tilt-in-space mechanism is usually preferred for pressure reduction to the buttocks over simply reclining the chair, since it avoids any friction that could also contribute to skin breakdown, as well as the muscle spasms that can be triggered by changes in body angle. This mechanism can be controlled by a joystick or even by head or chin movements. Some people use a "sip and puff" system, in which "puffing" on a straw enables the wheelchair to move in one direction and "sipping" in the other.

Proper positioning of the body in one's wheelchair is also crucial for preventing pressure sores. Most rehabilitation hospitals have specialized clinics devoted entirely to wheelchair evaluation and ordering. The appropriate wheelchair back-support system is crucial for ensuring the best posture, which will help prevent skin breakdown and pain. For example, leg rests and footplates need to be properly aligned so that they can support some of the body's weight and thereby relieve pressure on the buttocks. In addition, various types of wheelchair cushions are available to help evenly distribute pressure and provide protection against the chair's hard edges.

Since lying in bed adds pressure to the back of the head, tailbone, and heels, many people with SCI sleep on special mattresses filled with foam, air, or gel. Extra pillows can be used to provide additional padding to bony body parts and help maintain certain positions. Resting splints for feet minimize pressure on the heels. The recommendation for people in bed is to switch from one side to the other every two hours (though in reality, my patients have found it quite difficult to follow this routine at home without twenty-four-hour care).

Because other factors besides pressure contribute to skin breakdown, such as friction, it's important to keep all clothing and bed linen wrinkle-free. Furthermore, special care should be taken to avoid sliding when moving in bed, or dragging during transfers; if the person requires assistance, lifting is always preferable. Skin should be kept clean and dry, since moisture softens skin and makes it break down more easily. This requires close attention to hygiene, with regular bowel and bladder routines followed to prevent accidents, and any wet clothing changed immediately. Similarly, items that dry out skin should be avoided, including harsh soaps or alcohol-based products. Spasticity also needs to be managed, since muscle spasms can cause skin to rub against objects like clothing or bed sheets and lead to breakdown.

EAT WELL, LOOK HARD, KEEP CLEAN

Adequate nutrition, including vitamin and protein intake, is important for prevention as well as treatment of pressure ulcers.

The Agency for Healthcare Research and Quality (AHRQ) recommends that *all* individuals consume 1.0 to 1.25 grams of protein per kilogram of body weight daily. For example, a man who weighs 180 pounds needs to consume between 2.9 and 3.62 ounces of protein each day. When a pressure sore develops, however, the recommended amount of protein increases to 1.25 to 1.5 grams/kilogram per day (or 2.9 to 4.34 ounces for the same 180-pound man) to enhance healing. (Foods high in protein include fish, lean red meat, milk, eggs, and cheese.) Vitamins and minerals such as vitamins C, E, and zinc are also vital for wound healing. A well-balanced diet with appropriate iron supplementation prevents anemia (a decrease in red blood cells needed to carry oxygen to skin and soft tissue), another risk factor for poor skin healing. Smoking and alcohol should be avoided, since both habits not only increase the risk for developing pressure ulcers but also interfere with skin healing. Drinking enough (non-alcoholic and non-caffeinated) fluids such as water keeps the skin and soft tissue moist and flexible, and thus less likely to tear and break down.

Body weight is another important factor in skin care. Underweight people are at risk for excess pressure and skin damage, since they have less soft tissue to "cushion" their bony body parts. They also may lack the proper nutrition to maintain healthy skin. On the other hand, those who carry extra pounds may have limited mobility and a tougher time doing regular pressure relief. Their added weight may also make transfers and turning in bed quite challenging, increasing the chance that these maneuvers will result in friction, which can cause skin breakdown. Moreover, when people gain weight, the fit and alignment of their equipment, like wheelchairs and braces, must be reevaluated to look for new areas of pressure. All these issues underscore the importance of attention to weight control after spinal cord injury, especially with the resulting decrease in physical activity, which compounds a person's risk for obesity.

Overall, the most important principle in the treatment of pressure ulcers is early detection. As soon as someone notices any injury, that is, an area of skin that is red and does not blanch (similar to a first-degree burn or sunburn), prompt treatment is necessary. First and foremost, it is important to discover all possible contributing factors and develop an appropriate management plan. More specifically, pressure must be relieved, friction avoided, and any other underlying problems like incontinence, malnutrition, or smoking eliminated. All mattresses, splints, and seating systems should also be checked.

Optimal healing will occur only if a wound is clean. Any dead tissue present in a pressure ulcer must be removed, a process called "debridement" that can be done in several ways. *Sharp debridement* involves the use of a scalpel or scissors to remove the devitalized tissue. Wet-to-dry dressings are an example of *mechanical debridement,* in which gauze is moistened with saline, applied to the ulcer, and allowed to dry. When the dry dressing is later removed, any dead tissue that has attached to the gauze will be pulled away, leaving a clean ulcer base. Sometimes whirlpool treatments are used in conjunction with mechanical debridement, since the water helps loosen the dead tissue and makes it easier to remove. *Enzymatic debridement* uses commercially prepared chemicals to dissolve the unhealthy tissue, a method that can be slow and expensive. Lastly, in *autolytic debridement,* special dressings are placed over the ulcers to allow the body's own enzymes to clean the debris. This method requires frequent cleansing of the wound to wash out the unhealthy tissue, as well as close monitoring for infection.

When a pressure ulcer is clean, the most effective dressings are those that keep the ulcer bed moist and the surrounding tissue dry. The choice of dressing depends on many factors, including the depth, size, and location of the wound, the amount of drainage, and the cost and ease of use. The availability of different products varies from hospital to hospital and agency to agency. Once a treatment has been started, the wound should be closely watched for signs of healing. These include decreased size and drainage, the presence of new, pinkish tissue that forms along the edges of the ulcer and moves toward the center, or controlled bleeding, which indicates the presence of good circulation to the area. On the other hand, a person must seek immediate medical attention if the size or drainage of the ulcer increases, redness expands around the sore, foul-smelling or greenish drainage develops, or a fever occurs. If not properly treated, pressure ulcers can become a life-threatening condition and contribute to infections involving the blood, heart, or bone, and even amputations.

In addition to dressing changes, some clinicians recommend other specialized treatments for pressure ulcers to enhance healing. Electrical stimulation, for example, has been shown to increase the rate of healing for ulcers that do not respond to usual treatment. Hyperbaric oxygen, normothermic infrared therapy, and pulsed electromagnetic field energy treatment have each been proposed as beneficial in the management of pressure ulcers, yet there is no scientific evidence that they work.

A new adjunctive therapy, vacuum-assisted closure (VAC), has shown promise over the last decade in healing difficult wounds. This technique involves placing a foam sponge into the ulcer, connecting it to a drainage tube, and applying negative pressure to the wound. This increases blood flow to the ulcer, decreases surrounding swelling, and clears any bacteria present—all of which promote healing. Research has shown that ulcers managed with this type of treatment heal faster and with less discomfort than those treated with standard dressings alone.

Unfortunately, deeper pressure ulcers that will *not* heal on their own may require surgery. Different procedures are used, depending on the location and severity of the wound. Some involve skin grafts, while others require surgically moving muscle and skin together in sections, called flaps, to patch over the skin sore. All these operations, though quite diverse, maintain the same goals: to speed up healing, improve patient hygiene and appearance, and limit any complications.

Pain: Understanding and Handling It

There are many reasons that an individual might experience pain after becoming paralyzed. Soft tissue, muscles, or joints may be injured, or the spinal cord's pain pathways may malfunction. Certain medical illnesses can also cause various types of discomfort. In fact, studies have found that 33–95 percent of people with SCI face a heightened degree of pain during their lifetime. Most of my patients have developed this complication sometime in the first year post-injury, with certain groups more at risk than others—such as those with gunshot wounds. The good news, though, is that very few people report severe or persistent pain, and most find that their discomfort decreases over time.

It is often difficult for physicians to fully understand a patient's pain. Descriptions are always subjective, and people frequently have a hard time characterizing what they feel. Individuals also have different thresholds for pain; what is unbearable for one person may be completely manageable for another. As a result, pain is often difficult to diagnose, and there is no definitive test for its presence or severity. Although people often expect clinicians to take X-rays of their painful body parts, these studies show a problem only when it involves bones. A CT scan or MRI cannot be ordered for every pain complaint; yet when pain interferes with a person's everyday life and ability to function, it needs to be controlled and ideally cured. Physicians usually attempt to treat whatever seems to be the most likely cause first, and if that particular remedy does not work, the next most likely source is considered and a different management tried until the patient's discomfort is better.

Musculoskeletal Pain

Musculoskeletal pain is also called mechanical pain, and it is most frequently caused by damage to the ligaments, surrounding muscles, soft tissues, and bones. Although often dull and aching, this type of discomfort may also be sharp. It is usually worsened by activity and relieved with rest. It can stem from some kind of repetitive muscular activity, like using a manual wheelchair for extended periods; trauma; normal degenerative changes from aging; or other localized illnesses. Specific sources of this type of pain, several of which have already been discussed in this chapter, include spasticity, long bone fractures, muscle strains, heterotopic ossification, carpal tunnel syndrome, bursitis, tendonitis, complex regional pain syndrome (formerly known as reflex sympathetic dystrophy), infections, or tumors.

In people with SCI, mechanical pain most frequently involves the upper limbs. Because "the arms become the legs" after paralysis, shoulder discomfort commonly develops from this overuse of muscle and soft tissue. (The usual degeneration of joints that occurs as one ages also contributes to this kind of pain.) In addition, muscular imbalances put the extremities at increased risk for altered and excessive mechanical stress. The use of the upper limbs for wheelchair mobility, transfers, and pressure relief makes them prone to rotator cuff tears and bicipital tendonitis, for example. Although some studies have shown that individuals with paraplegia are most prone to shoulder problems, others claim that those with tetraplegia have just as much, if not more, discomfort. In my experience, upper-limb pain is a common complaint for both groups. The recommended treatment for these conditions is usually rest (accompanied by nonsteroidal anti-inflammatory medications), but this can be extremely challenging for a person with paraplegia who depends on his upper body for most of his physical activities. Once the acute pain is better, gentle range-of-motion exercises and strengthening can begin. Clinicians will also want to review how an individual transfers (or moves from place to place) to ensure that he or she is using proper body mechanics to reduce tissue strain and prevent recurrent injury.

Although carpal tunnel syndrome is actually a neurological disorder, it is described here under mechanical pain since it results from recurrent trauma to the hand and wrist, which can occur during wheelchair propulsion, transfers, and pressure relief. Manual wheelchair users put constant stress on their palms during these maneuvers, which can strain the median nerve that travels through a narrow canal in the wrist called the carpal tunnel. Burning and tingling in the thumb and first two fingers results and often intensifies at night. The longer it's been since a person's injury, the more common this condition becomes. Treatment again involves rest as well as splinting; pain medications are usually helpful, and steroid injections are frequently tried. Padded gloves should be used for wheelchair mobility to protect hands and wrists, and occupational therapy is often prescribed to correct poor technique or positioning. If these measures don't bring relief, surgery may be required. Some individuals also switch to a power wheelchair in later years to reduce the cumulative trauma to their wrists and shoulders.

Back or neck pain can be common in those who have had spinal fusions. During these surgeries, which are done to stabilize the vertebral column, spinal segments are made immobile; subsequently, higher stress is placed on adjacent segments and soft tissues. In the worst scenario, the spine eventually becomes unstable and additional surgery may be necessary. Moreover, if a person has limited range of motion at the hip owing to spasticity, contracture, or heterotopic ossification, the spine may be forced to work harder to maintain the sitting position—a process that can also result in mechanical back pain.

"Overuse" injuries may also occur in the lower extremities when certain muscles are forced to work double-time to compensate for others that are weak or paralyzed. In addition, uncontrolled spasticity in the hips, knees, or ankles may result in musculoskeletal pain that is best managed with stretching and proper positioning. Finally, degenerative changes involving the hip and pelvic joints that occur as part of the normal aging process can contribute to mechanical discomfort.

Neuropathic Pain

Neuropathic, or nerve, pain occurs as a result of damage to the central nervous system (the brain or spinal cord) or the peripheral nervous system (the outlying peripheral nerves). It is often difficult to tell exactly where the pain is coming from, but it is usually characterized by burning, tingling, shooting, stabbing, or stinging discomfort. People often use the terms "pins and needles," "twisting knife," and "electric shock-like" to describe it. Certain individuals tend to complain of neuropathic pain more frequently than others, including those disabled by gunshot wounds, individuals with incomplete injuries, and people with damage to the *cauda equina*. While this type of pain may begin soon after paralysis (often within the first year), its frequency and intensity usually diminish with time.

Although peripheral nerve problems like carpal tunnel syndrome represent one kind of neuropathic pain, the most bothersome type, known as central pain, stems from damage to the actual spinal cord itself. This usually involves both sides of the body, and includes the upper extremities, genitals, or, often, the entire body below the level of injury. Sometimes only the feet and hands are involved, called a "stocking glove" distribution. Body parts that cannot usually be felt by the person with SCI now become extremely painful when that part is touched. The discomfort is usually steady, but it can become more or less intense depending on factors like anxiety, fatigue, smoking, or the presence of other medical problems that occur below the level of injury. These can include a distended (overfull) bladder, constipation, pressure sore, or even an ingrown toenail.

The exact mechanism for neuropathic pain is unclear, but it is thought to be similar to the phantom pain experienced by amputees who still feel uncomfortable sensations from their lost limbs. Despite a missing body part or damaged spinal cord, the pain may stem from the sensory systems that remain intact and continue to generate messages that become abnormal and painful. Another possibility is that the spinal cord pathways that create and carry pain information may be impaired and more "excitable," sending mixed-up nerve messages that cause this discomfort. Maybe it is the pathways trying to reestablish connections—and if this is the case, neuropathic pain could actually be a *good* thing. Many theories have been postulated to explain this type of pain, but its exact mechanism remains poorly defined.

Visceral Pain

Visceral pain originates from damage, irritation, or enlargement of internal organs or their associated soft tissue structures. Examples include fecal impaction; bowel infarction or perforation; gall stones or kidney stones; appendicitis or pancreatitis; and bladder or kidney infections. For someone with SCI, the sensation to these organs changes and the discomfort (usually abdominal) associated with these medical conditions is often vague, dull, and difficult to locate.

For example, a perforated appendix can be just as painful as an abdominal muscle strain, depending on the amount of sensation a paralyzed individual has. While some people are able to point to the exact location of their pain, like the right lower abdomen in the case of appendicitis, others will only note right shoulder pain with the same condition. Because of their similar quality and location, some musculoskeletal and neuropathic sources of pain, such as abdominal wall spasticity, can easily be mistaken for visceral pain. Yet when someone has true visceral pain, there are usually other associated symptoms such as fever, increased abdominal muscle tone, and elevated blood pressure or heart rate that will help indicate the presence of a serious medical condition that warrants immediate attention.

Syringomyelia

Another important cause of pain after SCI is syringomyelia, or syrinx, which is a fluid-filled cavity that forms within the spinal cord and puts increasing pressure on the cord and its nerves. This complication affects 2–5 percent of people with traumatic spinal cord injuries; the onset is usually delayed, often until after the first year, though it can occur anytime—from two months post-injury to even decades later. People usually complain of intermittent pain, often at the site of their original injury and radiating to the neck or upper limbs, with a burning or dull, aching feeling (though some have reported sharp, electrical, or stabbing sensations). The discomfort may increase with coughing, sneezing, or straining, and many people also find that the level of their sensory loss rises. In addition, increased spasticity and weakness may occur.

The best way to diagnose this complication is with a spinal MRI. Treatment is controversial: some physicians recommend close monitoring only, while others advocate surgery to drain the fluid-filled cavity. The good news is that surgery has been shown to prevent further neurological damage and often lessens the pain.

Pain Treatment

The effective management of pain after paralysis requires close collaboration between the individual and his or her healthcare professional. Patience, cooperation, and ingenuity are essential for making an accurate diagnosis and selecting the best treatment strategy. Above all, the physician, in many cases a physiatrist, must rule out any serious conditions that could be the source of the pain.

The best initial approach to managing pain is always the least invasive (or most conservative). The mainstays of pain treatment and prevention include good nutrition and hydration, proper positioning and stretching exercises, ample physical activity to prevent weakness, and enough rest to stave off injury. People with paralysis must be aware of the potential factors that will contribute to their pain (for example, infection, pressure sores, smoking, uncontrolled spasticity) and learn how to prevent and manage them.

Because depression, stress, and fatigue will make pain worse, attention to a person's emotional well-being is critical. Supportive counseling, training in relaxation techniques, hypnosis, and biofeedback have all been shown to be helpful in managing pain. Individuals who remain active in their communities and involved with family and friends post-injury report much less pain than those who do not reach out, underscoring the importance of psychosocial factors. Often, participating in hobbies and social activities allows people to divert attention from any physical discomfort they may have.

At the very least, improving one's general well-being through therapeutic exercise will help to relieve pain. For mechanical pain, in particular, attention to proper range of motion, muscular imbalances, and correct posture in the form of physical and/ or occupational therapy can greatly increase comfort. Many people benefit from the use of heat, ice, or massage, as well as acupuncture. Others have found that transcutaneous electrical nerve stimulation (TENS), the stimulation of peripheral nerves using a small battery-operated unit with electrodes that is applied to the skin, is an effective means of easing pain.

Medications may become necessary when pain is disabling, limiting a person's everyday routine or interfering with sleep. The first-line agent for pain relief should always be acetaminophen or aspirin, depending on an individual's medical history. These medications carry minimal risk for side effects and are frequently effective pain relievers. Nonsteroidal anti-inflammatory drugs like ibuprofen or naproxen are also often used, especially during the early stages of musculoskeletal pain that results from overuse or trauma. These medications, however, must be taken cautiously, since gastrointestinal bleeding and kidney problems can occur.

When pain is so extreme that it can't be controlled with the drugs listed above, narcotics such as codeine or morphine may be needed. These analgesics are helpful in pain management, but they also present a dangerous potential for dependence and abuse and are thus best used for limited durations. Narcotics can also lead to constipation and drowsiness, side effects about which individuals should be forewarned.

For neuropathic pain, different types of medications are used, including the tricyclic antidepressants and various anticonvulsants. Although few studies have been conducted proving their definitive effectiveness, many individuals have found significant pain relief from the burning, stabbing discomfort of nerve-based pain using these agents. Such medications work by reducing the elimination of certain pain-relieving neurotransmitters in the bloodstream, thereby boosting their presence in the central nervous system and allowing them to "stay around" to work on alleviating pain. Unfortunately, many people who take the tricyclic antidepressants develop side effects such as dry mouth or bowel and bladder difficulties, even at the lower dose needed for pain control, and will often discontinue them. Anticonvulsants like gabapentin and topiramate, by contrast, have been generally well tolerated and continue to show increasing promise in the management of neuropathic pain.

Overall, when it comes to selecting the appropriate medication to treat pain, trial and error is the key. Patients must be aware of potential side effects and watch closely for adverse reactions. Despite all the studies and anecdotal experiences, it's clear that no one specific medication works for all types of pain or for all people.

When an individual's discomfort is localized and conservative measures have been exhausted, injections are another treatment option. More specifically, when nonsteroidal anti-inflammatory drugs have not helped or cannot be used, steroid injections into joints or soft tissue may provide rapid relief for pain caused by inflammation. Once the discomfort improves, the appropriate exercises and stretching can then be started. This is often the recommended course for subacromial bursitis or rotator cuff tendonitis, both of which affect the shoulder. In nerve blocks, another type of injection, chemicals like alcohol or phenol are used to destroy specific peripheral nerves and their "pain-causing" properties.

More recently, intramuscular injections of botulinum toxin (or Botox) have been successfully used to treat the mechanical pain associated with spasticity. Although side effects are few, the high cost—and the effort needed to make sure insurance companies provide coverage for the procedure—as well as the short duration of Botox's response (three to six months on average), may dissuade some people. This is especially true given that repeated injections are necessary to maintain results. Additionally, some people develop antibodies to the treatment, which makes the injections less effective in relieving pain as time goes on.

While various invasive surgeries have been used in the past to treat intractable pain in those with SCI, people now prefer more conservative measures, especially because these procedures often had disappointing results and were quite radical in nature. For example, surgeries called cordotomies were performed in the 1950s and 1960s and involved removing specific pain pathways of the spinal cord. These procedures ultimately had limited success, however, and frequently left individuals to develop even worse neuropathic pain months to years later. In the 1980s another procedure, the dorsal root entry zone (DREZ) ablation, was recommended for treating severe spinal cord injury pain, since it essentially destroyed the nerve cells that were thought to be the source of painful sensory information within the spinal cord. It, too, eventually fell out of favor when complications such as increased weakness and new sensory loss were noted.

As the examples in this chapter and the entire book show, people with spinal cord injury must grapple with challenges that go far beyond handling life in a wheelchair. Before my patients leave the rehab hospital I make sure they are educated about the various secondary illnesses and conditions described here, and I offer them reading material to reinforce what they've learned and give them something to consult after they've returned home. They are entering a much-anticipated phase of their recovery, but as a physician I want to make sure they are ready for any potential problems that may arise.

Just like those who have endured strokes, brain injuries, or other life-altering conditions, men, women, and children with paralysis remain at risk for potential complications long after their initial injury. Although the circumstances and obstacles will vary, the optimal strategy is always to gain full understanding of the situation, investigate the treatment options, and approach them head-on with determination and support from caregivers, family, and friends. Only in this way can a person work through all the issues that arise during recovery and continue on his or her path to the healthiest, most functional life possible after SCI.

APPENDIX

RESOURCES

SUGGESTED READING

ACKNOWLEDGMENTS

INDEX

Spinal Cord Injury by the Numbers

Approximately 11,000 people in the United States sustain traumatic spinal cord injuries each year, not including those who die at the scene of accidents. Although many states have government-sponsored registries that track such traumas, not all states use this kind of system, thus any such statistics must be considered estimates. Furthermore, since no organized system exists for reporting the incidence of non-traumatic injuries, paralysis that results from tumors, infections, surgical complications, and other causes is essentially excluded from the numbers. What we *do* know is that more people are living with spinal cord injuries today than ever before, an estimated 183,000 to 250,000 people in the United States alone. Better medical care and longer life expectancy, rather than an increased number of accidents, are behind these larger figures.

Traumatic spinal cord injuries primarily affect young adults, the group most prone to risk-taking behavior, according to demographics compiled between 1973 and 2003 by the NIDDR Spinal Cord Injury Model Systems of Care National Spinal Cord Injury Database. More than half of all such incidents (51.6 percent) occur in people aged sixteen to thirty, but with the graying of the baby boomer population, the average age at injury—now just over thirty-three years—has been rising, as has the proportion of those individuals who are older than sixty when paralyzed, usually as a result of falls. In all age groups, however, men are more often injured than women, at a rate of 4-to-1 overall. Caucasians represent the largest group of those with new injuries (66 percent), followed by African Americans (21 percent), Hispanic-Latinos (9.7 percent), and other groups including Native Americans, Eskimos, Asian-Pacific Islanders, and unknowns (3.5 percent).

The number one cause of traumatic spinal cord injury remains motor vehicle accidents, followed by falls, violence, and recreational sports activities. Despite the relatively high percentage of people paralyzed annually in car crashes, however, this statistic is on a downward trend as a result of air bags, mandatory seat-belt laws, reduced speed limits, and better auto design. Whereas every age group is involved to some extent in motor vehicle accidents, most people who become paralyzed from falls are predominantly at one of two age extremes, either the elderly or the very young. Diving accidents account for the most injuries among recreational sports, followed by (in order of frequency) snow skiing, football, surfing, horseback riding, and wrestling. Improvements in equipment and changes in rules regarding potentially hazardous tackles have helped reduce the number of injuries in football, while the removal of trampolines from schools in some states has likewise led to lower numbers in this activity. Interestingly, though the total number of spinal cord injuries in gymnastics is lower than in other sports, such injuries actually occur at a higher rate per athlete than injuries in football.

A far more challenging trend since the early 1970s is the growing number of injuries caused by acts of violence. Since these incidents disproportionately involve young African-American and Hispanic-Latino males living in the inner city, more attention has been given to establishing programs in urban areas that encourage non-violent methods of resolving conflict and safe recreational activities (such as organized late-night basketball leagues). But despite these efforts, and an overall decline in violence nationally since a peak in the mid-1990s, the problem of spinal cord injuries acquired through gunshot wounds and stabbings persists.

Given the young age at which most people become paralyzed, it is no surprise that the majority of them are single at the time. Once individuals become spinal cord injured, they are also less likely to marry—and more likely to divorce if they do find a spouse—than the general population. (Chapter 7, "Couples and Relationship Issues," touches more on this subject. However, this analysis does not factor in same-sex couples that consist of one or two SCI partners.) In terms of employment, many of those who become paralyzed previously worked in traditionally "blue-collar" jobs, making it more difficult for them to return to work. As a group, only 60.2 percent of those injured received at least a high school diploma, and very few hold higher degrees. (More details about return-to-work issues are discussed in Chapter 4, "Back to Productivity.")

In addition, though a majority of those aged sixteen to fifty-nine are employed at the time of injury, 18.7 percent of new injuries overall are incurred by people out of work. Surprisingly, the percentage of people with paraplegia who are able to return to the workforce is only slightly higher than that of people with tetraplegia. Although the determination and support system an individual possesses always play a key role in a possible return to work, the severity of a person's disability is nonetheless directly proportional to his or her chances for reemployment.

With improvements in health care, people with SCI continue to live longer, though their life expectancy is still shorter than that of the general population. Although the majority of deaths occur in the first year post-injury, it is important to note that this statistic pertains largely to those who have had the most severe injuries or are of advanced age. With each subsequent year of survival, the risk of premature death declines steadily. Whereas thirty years ago the leading cause of death for paralyzed individuals was kidney disease, today respiratory illnesses (like pneumonia) and other infections are most often to blame. This change is undoubtedly due to vastly improved follow-up medical care, as well as to the greater number of people surviving with tetraplegia and extensive injuries.

In terms of level of injury, people with tetraplegia are more likely to die from pneumonia, while those with paraplegia usually die from heart disease, overwhelming infection (septicemia), and suicide. Yet now, as a result of advances in the medical care of people with spinal cord injury, the majority of those with SCI have a higher chance than ever of dying from the very same causes as the general population: heart disease and cancer.

Resources

Access for Disabled Americans
A nonprofit corporation helping people with disabilities live and function in an accessible, barrier-free environment by providing assistance with employment, education, home and workplace accessibility, travel opportunities, and transportation.
3685 Mt. Diablo Blvd., No. 300
Lafayette, CA 94549
Office: 925-284-6444
Fax: 925-284-6448
www.accessfordisabled.com

Alliance for Technology Access (ATA)
National network of community-based resource centers in many states that provide information and support services to children and adults with disabilities, with the goal of increasing their use of assistive and information technologies.
1304 Southpoint Blvd., Suite 240
Petaluma, CA 94954
Phone: 707-778-3011
TTY: 707-778-3015
Fax: 707-765-2080
www.ataccess.org

American Academy of Physical Medicine and Rehabilitation (AAPM&R)

A national medical society representing more than 7,000 physicians (called physiatrists) who are specialists in the field of physical medicine and rehabilitation. Great search feature on website allows users to find contact information on all member physiatrists by region and state.

330 North Wabash Ave., Suite 2500
Chicago, IL 60611-7617
Phone: 312-464-9700
Fax: 312-464-0227
www.aapmr.org

American Association of Spinal Cord Injury Psychologists and Social Workers (AASCIPSW)

A networking group that seeks to advance, encourage, and improve psychosocial care of people with SCI, in part by promoting education and research.

75-20 Astoria Blvd.
Jackson Heights, NY 11370
Phone: 718-803-3782
Fax: 718-803-0414
www.aascipsw.org

American Spinal Injury Association (ASIA)

A multidisciplinary organization of physicians, researchers, allied health professionals, and advocates involved in spinal cord injury care, research, and prevention. ASIA is strongly focused on educating healthcare professionals, patients, and families about SCI and its consequences.

2020 Peachtree Rd., NW
Atlanta, GA 30309
Phone: 404-355-9772
Fax: 404-355-1826
www.asia-spinalinjury.org

Christopher and Dana Reeve Paralysis Resource Center (PRC)

An organization that serves as a comprehensive, national source of information for people living with paralysis and their caregivers to promote health, foster involvement in the community, and improve quality of life. Robust website includes detailed information on everything from modifying a home to parenting with a disability to maintaining one's health, with links to other related sites.

Short Hills Plaza
636 Morris Turnpike, Suite No. 3A
Short Hills, NJ 07078
Phone: 800-539-7309
(Information specialists available daily from 9 A.M. to 8 P.M. Eastern Standard Time)
www.paralysis.org

National Spinal Cord Injury Association (NSCIA)

The nation's oldest and largest civilian organization dedicated to improving the quality of life for people with spinal cord injuries and their loved ones. The association has a terrific peer support network and resource center, as well as a website featuring an "A to Z" resource guide, back issues of various NSCIA publications, and links to research and clinical updates.

6701 Democracy Blvd., Suite 300-9
Bethesda, MD 20817
Phone (helpline): 800-962-9629
Voicemail: 301-214-4006
Fax: 301-990-0445
www.spinalcord.org

Paralyzed Veterans of America (PVA)

The only congressionally chartered veterans organization dedicated solely to serving the needs of veterans with SCI. The PVA is a leading advocate for health care, research and education, veterans' benefits and rights, sports programs, disability rights, and accessibility issues including the removal of architectural barriers.

National Headquarters
801 Eighteenth St., NW
Washington, DC 20006-3517
Phone: 800-424-8200
www.pva.org

Spinal Cord Injury Information Network
Comprehensive online source of SCI information and resources
gathered from various academic rehab centers, organizations, agencies, and more. Website has extensive links to other disability-related
sites and details on various publications.
UAB Model SCI System
Office of Research Services
619 19th St. South, SRC 529
Birmingham, AL 35249-7330
Phone: 205-934-3283
www.spinalcord.uab.edu

CAREGIVER ORGANIZATIONS

Canine Companions for Independence (CCI)
Nonprofit organization that provides highly trained assistance dogs
and ongoing support to children and adults with disabilities.
National Headquarters and Northwest Regional Center
2965 Dutton Ave.
P.O. Box 446
Santa Rosa, CA 95402-0446
Phone: 707-577-1700
TTY: 707-577-1756
www.caninecompanions.org

Family Caregiver Alliance (FCA)
Often described as a "one-stop shopping center for caregivers," FCA
offers a wide array of services and publications based on caregiver
needs and offers programs at the local, state, and national level.

180 Montgomery St., Suite 1100
San Francisco, CA 94104
Phone: 800-445-8106
Fax: 415-434-3508
www.caregiver.org

National Family Caregivers Association (NFCA)

Organization that educates, supports, and empowers those who care for loved ones with a chronic illness or disability or the challenges of old age. NFCA reaches across the boundaries of diagnoses, relationships, and life stages to address the common needs and concerns of all family caregivers.
10400 Connecticut Ave., Suite 500
Kensington, MD 20895-3944
Toll Free: 800-896-3650
Phone: 301-942-6430
Fax: 301-942-2302
www.nfcacares.org

Well Spouse Association (WSA)

National, not-for-profit membership organization that supports wives, husbands, and partners of the chronically ill and/or disabled. Well Spouse support groups meet monthly and set up letter writing "round robins" to help members who are largely isolated at home caring for loved ones.
63 West Main St., Suite H
Freehold, NJ 07728
Phone: 800-838-0879
Fax: 732-577-8644
www.wellspouse.org

CHILDREN AND TEENS WITH DISABILITIES

National Dissemination Center for Children with Disabilities (NICHCY)

A central source of bilingual (English, Spanish) information on disabilities in infants, toddlers, children, and teens, with focus on IDEA (the law authorizing special education); the No Child Left Behind law (as it relates to children with disabilities); and research-based information on effective educational practices.

P.O. Box 1492
Washington, DC 20013
Phone: 800-695-0285
Fax: 202-884-8441
www.nichcy.org

Winners on Wheels (WOW)

National network of programs designed specifically for children with disabilities. WOW provides an innovative online learning environment that promotes academic, social, and emotional development so kids in wheelchairs can gain skills and experiences to further their quality of life and independence.

302 E. Church St.
Lewisville, TX 75057
Phone: 800-WOW-TALK (969-8255)
Fax: 559-291-3386
www.wowusa.com

EMPLOYMENT SERVICES, PROGRAMS, AND RESOURCES

American Congress of Community Supports and Employment Services (ACCSES)

A national nonprofit organization that uses a strong network of state vocational rehabilitation services and a grassroots presence on Capitol Hill to help maximize employment opportunities and independent living for individuals with mental and physical disabilities.

1501 M St., NW, 7th floor
Washington, DC 20005
Phone: 202-466-3355
Fax: 202-466-7571
www.accses.org

Americans with Disabilities Act (ADA) Home Page

Comprehensive guide to the landmark 1991 disability ruling, including a primer in disability rights law, information on ADA standards for businesses and accessible design, and links to other resources regarding rights of people with disabilities.

U.S. Department of Justice

950 Pennsylvania Ave., NW

Civil Rights Division

Disability Rights Section—NYA

Washington, DC 20530

Phone: 800-514-0301

TTY: 800-514-0383

Fax: 202-307-1198

www.usdoj.gov/crt/ada

Disabled Businesspersons Association

A charitable organization dedicated to helping enterprising individuals with disabilities maximize their potential in the business world, and to working with vocational and government organizations to encourage and increase the participation of disabled people in the workforce.

San Diego State University–Interwork Institute

5950 Hardy Ave., Suite 112

San Diego, CA 92182-5313

Phone: 619-594-8805

Fax: 619-594-4208

www.disabledbusiness.com

Social Security Administration

Federal agency administering the Social Security Disability Insurance (SSDI) and Supplemental Security Income (SSI) programs, which offer benefits to disabled individuals on the basis of prior work experience (SSDI) or financial need (SSI).

Office of Public Inquiries
Windsor Park Building
6401 Security Blvd.
Baltimore, MD 21235
Phone: 800-772-1213
TTY: 800-325-0778
www.ssa.gov

The Work Site (Social Security Online)

Provides links to vocational rehabilitation programs in all fifty states
and other U.S. territories. Also supplies links to information about
the safety net of work incentives that Social Security beneficiaries can
use to keep their cash benefits and health insurance coverage as they
begin working and progress in employment.
www.ssa.gov/work/ServiceProviders/rehabproviders

ASSISTIVE TECHNOLOGY AND EQUIPMENT

AbleData

A federally funded database providing information on assistive technology and rehabilitation equipment from domestic and international sources. Offers detailed product descriptions, including price
and company information, as well as toll-free quick reference and referral services and training workshops.
8630 Fenton St., Suite 930
Silver Spring, MD 20910
Phone: 800-227-0216
TTY: 301-608-8912
Fax: 301-608-8958
www.abledata.com

Sammons Preston Rolyan

Company offering extensive online and paper catalogs of mobility
aides and equipment to assist with activities of daily living. Ordering
assistance available twenty-four hours a day.

P.O. Box 5071
Bolingbrook, IL 60440-5071
Phone: 800-323-5547
Fax: 800-547-4333
www.sammonspreston.com

PARENTING WITH A DISABILITY

Through the Looking Glass (TLG)

A nonprofit, community-based organization that grew out of the independent living movement. TLG has pioneered research, training,
and services for families in which a child, parent, or grandparent has
a disability or medical issue. TLG's National Resource Center for Parents with Disabilities provides information, referrals, publications,
training, and consultations on parenting with a disability, and also
publishes a popular guide on adaptive babycare equipment.
2198 Sixth St., Suite 100
Berkeley, CA 94710-2204
Phone: 800-644-2666
TTY: 800-804-1616
Local: 510-848-1112
Fax: 510-848-4445
www.lookingglass.org

RECREATION AND SPORTS

Access-Able Travel Source

Website devoted to helping individuals with disabilities locate travel
resources, as well as links to travel agencies with expertise in meeting
the needs of disabled travelers. Great "travel tales" from fellow vaca-
tioners.
P. O. Box 1796
Wheat Ridge, CO 80034
Phone: 303-232-2979
Fax: 303-239-8486
www.access-able.com

Disabled Sports USA

Organization that offers nationwide sports rehabilitation programs
to anyone with a permanent disability. Activities include winter skiing, water sports, summer and winter competitions, fitness, and special sports events. Nationwide chapter networks available in every region of the United States.

451 Hungerford Dr., Suite 100
Rockville, MD 20850
Phone: 301-217-0960
Fax: 301-217-0968
www.dsusa.org

Flying Wheels Travel
(a division of Travel Headquarters, Inc.)

A full-service agency specializing in travel for persons with
disabilities. Provides escorted tours outside the United States,
mainly to Europe and the Middle East. Offers worldwide cruises
on both an individual and an escorted basis, and customized itin-
eraries for disabled travelers with able-bodied companions worldwide.

143 W. Bridge St.
Owatonna, MN 55060
Phone: 507-451-5005
Fax: 507-451-1685
www.flyingwheelstravel.com

National Wheelchair Poolplayers Association, Inc. (NWPA)

The governing body for all organized wheelchair pool. NWPA holds
tournaments nationwide and maintains a website that provides
schedule information and an online store.

820 Coastal Beach Rd.
Henderson, NV 89002
www.nwpainc.org

North American Riding for the Handicapped Association (NARHA)
Organization that promotes equine-facilitated therapy and activity
programs in the United States and Canada, with more than 650 pro-
gram centers serving some 30,000 individuals with disabilities.
P.O. Box 33150
Denver, CO 80233
Phone: 800-369-7433
Fax: 303-252-4610
www.narha.org

United States Quad Rugby Association
Comprehensive website providing information on the wheelchair
sport popularized in the movie *Murderball,* including rules, tourna-
ment resources and results, links to clinics, and a chat room.
www.quadrugby.com

SEXUALITY

Sexual Health Network
Website dedicated to providing easy access to education, support, and
other resources related to sexuality, including comprehensive section
on sex after SCI.
3 Mayflower Lane
Shelton, CT 06484
www.sexualhealth.com

Suggested Reading

CHAPTER 1: INTRODUCTION TO SPINAL CORD INJURY

Jackson, A. B., et al. "A Demographic Profile of New Traumatic Spinal Cord Injuries: Change and Stability over Thirty Years," *Archives of Physical Medicine and Rehabilitation*, vol. 85, Nov. 2004 (pp. 1740–1748).

Meade, M., et al. "Race, Employment, and Spinal Cord Injury," *Archives of Physical Medicine and Rehabilitation*, vol. 85, Nov. 2004 (pp. 1782–1792).

Stover, S., J. DeLisa, and G. Whiteneck. *Spinal Cord Injury—Clinical Outcomes from the Model Systems*. Gaithersburg, MD: Aspen Publishers, 1995 (pp. 25–52).

CHAPTER 2: EARLY DAYS; AND CHAPTER 3: ADJUSTING TO SCI

Caplan, B., and K. Reidy. "Staff-Patient-Family Conflicts in Rehabilitation: Sources and Solutions," *Topics in Spinal Cord Injury Rehabilitation*, 2, 1996 (pp. 21–33).

Caplan, B., and J. Schecter. "Denial and Depression in Disabling Illness," in B. Caplan, ed., *Rehabilitation Psychology Desk Reference*. Rockville, MD: Aspen Publishers, 1987.

Cushman, L. A., and M. Dijkers. "Depressed Mood during Rehabilitation of Persons with Spinal Cord Injury," *Journal of Rehabilitation*, 2, 1991 (pp. 35–38).

Devivo, M. J., et al. "Suicide Following Spinal Cord Injury," *Paraplegia*, 29, 1991 (pp. 625–627).

Frank, R., et al. "Depression after Spinal Cord Injury: Is It Necessary?" *Clinical Psychology Review*, 7, 1987 (pp. 611–630).

Frank, R., and T. Elliott. "Life Stress and Psychologic Adjustment Following Spinal Cord Injury," *Archives of Physical Medicine and Rehabilitation*, 68, 1987 (pp. 344–347).

Furnham, A., and R. Thompson. "Actual and Perceived Attitudes of Wheelchair Users," *Counseling Psychology Quarterly*, 7, 1994 (pp. 35–51).

Hammell, K. W. "Psychological and Sociological Theories concerning Adjustment to Traumatic Spinal Cord Injury: The Implications for Rehabilitation," *Paraplegia*, 30, 1992 (pp. 317–326).

Heinemann, A. W., B. D. Mamott, and S. Schnoll. "Substance Use by Persons with Recent Spinal Cord Injury," *Rehabilitation Psychology*, 35 (4), 1990 (pp. 217–228).

McLeod, M. B. "Self-Neglect of Spinal Injured Patients," *Paraplegia*, 26, 1988 (pp. 340–348).

Moore, A. D., and D. R. Patterson. "Psychological Intervention with Spinal Cord Injured Patients: Promoting Control out of Dependence," *SCI Psychosocial Process*, 6 (1), Feb. 1993 (pp. 2–8).

Morris, J. "Spinal Injury and Psychotherapy: A Treatment Philosophy," in *Spinal Cord Injury: Medical Management and Rehabilitation* (4th ed.), ed. G. Yarkony. Gaithersburg, MD: Aspen Publishers, 1994 (pp. 223–231).

Olkin, R. "The Minority Model of Disability," *What Psychotherapists Should Know about Disability*. New York: Guilford Press, 1999 (pp. 24–54).

Woodbury, B. "Psychological Adjustment to Spinal Cord Injury: A Literature Review, 1950–1977," *Rehabilitation Psychology*, 25, 1978 (pp. 119–134).

CHAPTER 4: BACK TO PRODUCTIVITY

Chapin, M., and D. Kewman. "Factors Affecting Employment Following Spinal Cord Injury: A Qualitative Study," *Rehabilitation Psychology*, 46 (4), 2001 (400–416).

Kahn, P., and R. C. Kahn. "Quads at Work," *New Mobility* magazine, Feb. 2001 (pp. 40–42).

Krause, J. S. "Employment after Spinal Cord Injury: Transition and Life Adjustment," *Rehabilitation Counseling Bulletin,* 39, 1996 (pp. 244–255).

———. "The Relationship between Productivity and Adjustment Following Spinal Cord Injury, *Rehabilitation Counseling Bulletin,* 33, 1990 (pp. 188–199).

Krause, J. S., et al. "Employment after Spinal Cord Injury: An Analysis of Cases from the Model Spinal Cord Injury System," *Archives of Physical Medicine and Rehabilitation,* 80, 1999 (pp. 1492–1500).

Sukiennik, G. "Eight Years after Accident, Travis Roy Taking on New Challenges," *Portland Press Herald,* Jan. 10, 2004.

Tomassen, P. C. D., M. W. M. Post, and F. W. A. Van Asbeck. "Return to Work after Spinal Cord Injury," *Spinal Cord,* 38, 2000 (pp. 51–55).

Treischmann, R. B. *Spinal Cord Injuries: Psychological, Social, and Vocational Rehabilitation* (2nd ed.). New York: Demos Publishing, 1987.

CHAPTER 5: DATING AFTER SCI; AND CHAPTER 6: SEXUAL FUNCTION AFTER SCI

Derry, F. A., et al. "Efficacy and Safety of Oral Sildenafil (Viagra) in Men with Erectile Dysfunction Caused by Spinal Cord Injury," *Neurology,* 51, 1998 (pp. 1629–1633).

Fisher, T. L., et al. "Sexual Health after Spinal Cord Injury: A Longitudinal Study," *Archives of Physical Medicine and Rehabilitation,* 83, 2002 (p. 8).

Geiger, R. C., "Neurophysiology of Sexual Response in Spinal Cord Injury," *Sexuality Disability,* 2, 1979 (pp. 257–265).

Goldstein, I., et al. "Oral Sildenafil in the Treatment of Erectile Dysfunction," *New England Journal of Medicine,* 338 (20), 1998 (pp. 1397–1404).

Green, B. G., et al. "Complications of Penile Implants in Spinal Cord

Injured Patients," *Topics in Spinal Cord Injury Rehabilitation*, 1 (2), 1995 (pp. 44–52).

Kreuter, M., et al. "Sexual Adjustment after Spinal Cord Injury (SCI) Focusing on Partner Experiences," *Paraplegia*, 32, 1994a (pp. 225–235).

————. "Sexual Adjustment after Spinal Cord Injury—Comparison of Partner Experiences in Pre- and Post-Injury Relationships," *Paraplegia*, 32, 1994b (pp. 759–770).

Mooney, T. O., T. M. Cole, and R. A. Chilgren. *Sexual Options for Paraplegics and Quadriplegics*. Boston: Little Brown, 1975.

Olkin, R. "Dating, Romance, and Sexuality," in *What Psychotherapists Should Know about Disability*. New York: Guilford Press, 1999 (pp. 224–254).

Sipski, M. L., and C. J. Alexander. *Sexual Function in People with Disability and Chronic Illness*. Gaithersburg, MD: Aspen Publishing, 1997.

Sipski, M. L., C. J. Alexander, and R. C. Rosen. "Orgasm in Women with Spinal Cord Injuries: A Laboratory-Based Assessment," *Archives of Physical Medicine and Rehabilitation*, 756, 1995 (pp. 1097–1102).

————. "Physiologic Parameters Associated with Psychogenic Sexual Arousal in Women with Complete Spinal Cord Injuries," *Archives of Physical Medicine and Rehabilitation*, 76, 1995 (pp. 811–818).

————. "Physiologic Parameters Associated with Sexual Arousal in Women with Incomplete Spinal Cord Injuries," *Archives of Physical Medicine and Rehabilitation*, 78, 1997 (pp. 305–313).

White, M. J., et al. "Sexual Activities, Concerns, and Interests of Men with Spinal Cord Injury," *American Journal of Physical Medicine and Rehabilitation*, 71, 1992 (pp. 225–231).

————. "Sexual Activities, Concerns, and Interests of Women with Spinal Cord Injury Living in the Community," *American Journal of Physical Medicine and Rehabilitation*, 72, 1993 (pp. 372–378).

CHAPTER 7: COUPLES AND RELATIONSHIP ISSUES

Byzek, J. "Committed Couples," *New Mobility*, Feb.–March 2001.

Corbet, B., J. Dobbs, and B. Bonin, eds. "Should a Spouse Do the

Care?" *Spinal Network: The Total Wheelchair Resource Book* (3rd ed.). Santa Monica, CA: Nine Lives Press, 2002 (p. 377).

Crewe, N. "Spousal Relationships and Disability," in F. P. Haseltine, S. Cole, and D. Gray, eds., *Reproductive Issues for Persons with Physical Disabilities*. Baltimore: Brookes, 1993.

Crewe, N. M., G. T. Athelstan, and J. Krumberger. "Spinal Cord Injury: A Comparison of Pre-Injury and Post-Injury Marriages," *Archives of Physical Medicine and Rehabilitation*, 60, 1979 (pp. 252–256).

Crewe, N. M., and J. S. Krause. "Marital Relationships and Spinal Cord Injury," *Archives of Physical Medicine and Rehabilitation*, 69, 1988 (pp. 435–438).

Decker, S. D., R. Schulz, and D. Wood. "Determinants of Well-Being in Primary Caregivers of Spinal Cord Injured Persons, *Rehabilitation Nursing*, 14, 1989 (pp. 6–8).

Devivo, M., and P. Fine. "Spinal Cord Injury: Its Short-Term Impact on Marital Status," *Archives of Physical Medicine and Rehabilitation*, 66, 1985 (pp. 501–504).

Devivo, M., et al. "Outcomes of Post–Spinal Cord Injury Marriages," *Archives of Physical Medicine and Rehabilitation*, 76, 1995 (pp. 130–138).

El Ghatit, A. A., and R. W. Hanson. "Marriage and Divorce after Spinal Cord Injury," *Archives of Physical Medicine and Rehabilitation*, 57, 1976 (pp. 470–472).

Elliott, T. R., R. M. Shewchuk, and J. S. Richards. "Family Caregiver Social Problem-Solving Abilities and Adjustment During the Initial Year of the Caregiving Role," *Journal of Counseling Psychology*, 48 (2), 2001 (pp. 223–232).

Holicky, R. "A Labor of Love—Beating Stress in Longterm Caregiving," *New Mobility*, June 2000.

Kreuter, M. "Spinal Cord Injury and Partner Relationships," *Spinal Cord*, 38, 2000 (pp. 2–6).

Ludwig, E. G., and J. Collette. "Disability, Dependency, and Conjugal Roles," *Journal of Marriage and the Family*, 31, 1969 (pp. 736–739).

McNeff, E. A. "Issues for the Partner of the Person with a Disability," in M. L. Sipski and C. J. Alexander, *Sexual Function in People with Disability and Chronic Illness.* Gaithersburg, MD: Aspen Publishing, 1997.

Olkin, R. "Families with Disability," In *What Psychotherapists Should Know about Disability.* New York: Guilford Press, 1999 (pp. 90–136).

Palmer, S., K. H. Kriegsman, and J. B. Palmer. *Spinal Cord Injury—A Guide for Living.* Baltimore: Johns Hopkins University Press, 2000.

Power, P. W., and A. Dell Orto. *Role of the Family in the Rehabilitation of the Physically Disabled.* Baltimore: University Park Press, 1980 (pp. 145–171).

Rolland, J. "In Sickness and in Health: The Impact of Illness on Couples' Relationships," *Journal of Marital and Family Therapy,* 4–920, 1994 (pp. 327–348).

Senelick, R., M.D., with K. Dougherty. *The Spinal Cord Injury Handbook for Patients and Their Families.* HealthSouth Press, 1998 (pp. 114–120).

"Sex and Disabilities," Part 2 of 4, *accessibility.com.au*—The disability information resource. We Media Inc., May 2000.

Tepper, M. S. "What Does Your Partner Find Sexy about Your Disability?" *Sexualhealth.com,* April 25, 2002.

Urey, J., and S. Henggler. "Marital Adjustment Following Spinal Cord Injury," *Archives of Physical Medicine and Rehabilitation,* 68, 1987 (pp. 69–74).

Weitzenkamp, B. A., et al. "Spouses of SCI Survivors: The Added Impact of Caregiving," *Archives of Physical Medicine and Rehabilitation,* 78, August 1997 (pp. 822–827).

Zahn, M. A. "Incapacity, Impotence, and Invisible Impairment: Their Effects upon Interpersonal Relations," *Journal of Health and Social Behavior,* 14, 1973 (pp. 115–123).

CHAPTER 8: FERTILITY AND PREGNANCY

Amador, M. J., C. M. Lynne, and N. L. Brackett. *A Guide and Resource Directory to Male Fertility Following Spinal Cord Injury/Dysfunction.* Miami Project to Cure Paralysis, 2000. (Funded by the Paralyzed Veterans of America SCI Education and Training Foundation.)

Baker, E. R., and D. D. Cardenas. "Pregnancy in Spinal Cord Injured Women," *Archives of Physical Medicine and Rehabilitation*, 77, 1996 (pp. 501–507).

Baker, E. R., D. D. Cardenas, and T. J. Benedetti. "Risks Associated with Pregnancy in Spinal Cord Injured Women," *Obstetrics and Gynecology*, 80, 1992 (pp. 425–428).

Beckerman, H., J. Becher, and G. J. Lankhorst. "The Effectiveness of Vibratory Stimulation in Anejaculatory Men with Spinal Cord Injury," Review Article, *Paraplegia*, 31, 1993 (pp. 689–699).

Brackett, N. L., M. S. Nash, and C. M. Lynne. "Male Fertility Following Spinal Cord Injury: Facts and Fiction," *Physical Therapy*, 76 (11), 1996 (pp. 1225–1228).

Brackett, N. L., R. P. Padron, and C. M. Lynne. "Semen Quality of Spinal Cord Injured Men Is Better When Obtained by Vibratory Stimulation v. Electroejaculation," *Journal of Urology*, 157, 1997 (pp. 152–156).

Cross, L. L., et al. "Pregnancy, Labor, Delivery Post Spinal Cord Injury," *Paraplegia*, 30, 1992 (pp. 890–902).

Linsenmeyer, T. A. "Male Infertility Following Spinal Cord Injury," *Journal of the American Paraplegia Society*, 14 (3), 1991 (pp. 116–120).

Lochner-Ernst, D., B. Mandulka, G. Kramer, and M. Stohrer, "Conservative and surgical semen retrieval in patients with Spinal Cord Injury," *Spinal Cord*, 35 (7), 1997 (pp. 463–468).

Matthews, G. J., T. A. Gardner, and J. F. Eid. "IVF Improves Pregnancy Rates for Sperm Obtained by Rectal Probe Ejaculation," *Journal of Urology*, 155 (6), 1996 (pp. 1934–1937).

Ohl, D. A., et al. "Predictions of Success in Electoejaculation of Spinal Cord Injured Men," *Journal of Urology*, 142, 1989 (pp. 1483–1486).

Seager, S. W. J., and L. S. Halstead. "Fertility Options and Success after Spinal Cord Injury," *Urology Clinical North America*, 20 (3), 1993 (pp. 543–548).

Sipski, M. L., and C. J. Alexander. *Sexual Function in People with Dis-*

ability and Chronic Illness. Gaithersburg, MD: Aspen Publishing, 1997.

Yarkony, G. M., and D. Chen. "Sexuality in Patients with Spinal Cord Injury," *Physical Medicine and Rehabilitation: State of the Art Reviews* 9 (2), June 1995 (pp. 325–344).

CHAPTER 9: PARENTING WITH SCI

Alexander, C. J., K. Hwang, and M. Sipski. "Mothers with Spinal Cord Injures: Impact on Marital, Family, and Children's Adjustment," *Archives of Physical Medicine and Rehabilitation,* 83 (1), 2002 (pp. 24–30).

Buck, F. M., and G. W. Hohmann. "Child Adjustment as Related to Severity of Paternal Disability, *Archives of Physical Medicine and Rehabilitation,* 63, 1982 (pp. 249–253).

———. "Personality, Behavior, Values, and Family Relations of Children of Fathers with Spinal Cord Injury," *Archives of Physical Medicine and Rehabilitation,* 62, 1981 (pp. 432–438).

Centre for Independent Living in Toronto (CILT) (assorted articles). Parenting Network's Parenting Bulletin, 1990–2005.

Crawford, N. "Parenting with a Disability: The Last Frontier," *Monitor on Psychology,* May 2003.

Gilmer, T. "The Purcells: A World of 9,000 Things," *New Mobility,* August 2000 (pp. 31–33).

Kirshblum, S., D. Campagnolo, and J. DeLisa, eds. *Spinal Cord Medicine.* Philadelphia: Lippincott Williams and Wilkins, 2002.

Olkin, R. *What Psychotherapists Should Know about Disability.* New York: Guilford Press, 1999.

Pischke, M. E. "Parenting with a Disability," *Sexuality Disability,* 11, 1993 (pp. 207–210).

Prilleltensky, O. *Motherhood and Disability: Children and Choices.* New York: Palgrave/MacMillan, 2004.

Rintala, D. H., L. Herson, and T. Hudler-Hull. "Comparison of Parenting Styles of Persons with and without Spinal Cord Injury and Their Children's Social Competence and Behavior Problems," *Journal of Spinal Cord Medicine,* 23 (4), Winter 2000 (pp. 244–256).

Samuels, R. "The Hockenberrys: A Family Portrait," *New Mobility,* August 2002 (pp. 26–30).

Tuleja, C., and A. DeMoss. "Babycare Assistive Technology," *Technology and Disability,* 11, 1991 (pp. 71–78).

Tuleja, C., et al. "Continuation of Adaptive Parenting Equipment Development," Through the Looking Glass's National Resource Center for Parents with Disabilities. NIDRR grant number H133B.30076, final report: January 1998.

Vensand, K., et al. *Adaptive Baby Care Equipment: Guidelines, Prototypes, and Resources.* Berkeley, CA: Through the Looking Glass, 2000.

CHAPTER 10: CHILDREN AND ADOLESCENTS WITH SCI

Belkin, D. "The Last Shot," *Boston Globe Magazine,* Aug. 1, 2004.

Betz, R. R., and M. J. Mulcahey, eds. *The Child with a Spinal Cord Injury.* Rosemont, IL: American Academy of Orthopedic Surgeons, 1996.

Dell Orto, A. E., and P. W. Power. "Impact of Disability/Illness on the Child," from *Role of the Family in the Rehabilitation of the Physically Disabled.* Baltimore: University Park Press, 1980.

Kremetz, J. *How It Feels to Live with a Physical Disability.* New York: Simon and Schuster, 1992.

Lammertse, D., A. B. Jackson, and M. L. Sipski. "Research from the Model Spinal Cord Injury Systems: Findings from the Current Five-Year Grant Cycle," *Archives of Physical Medicine and Rehabilitation,* vol. 85, no. 11, Nov. 2004.

McCollum, A. T. "Grieving Over the Lost Dream," from *The Disabled Child and Family: An Exceptional Parent Reader,* M. Schleifer and S. D. Klein, eds. Boston, MA: Exceptional Parents Press, 1985.

Palmer, S., K. H. Kreigsman, and J. Palmer. *Spinal Cord Injury—A Guide for Living.* Baltimore: Johns Hopkins University Press, 2000 (esp. Chap. II-5, "Focus on the Family").

Panzarino, C., and M. Lash. *Rebecca Finds a New Way: How Kids Learn, Play, and Live with Spinal Cord Injuries and Illnesses.* Woburn, MA: National Spinal Cord Injury Association, 1994.

Rousso, M. "Fostering Healthy Self-Esteem," from *The Disabled Child and Family: An Exceptional Parent Reader,* M. Schleifer and S. D. Klein, eds. Boston, MA: Exceptional Parents Press.

Tao, C. "Teens with Spinal Cord Injuries," *Washington Times,* June 21, 2005; republished online at the Spinal Cord Injury Zone (www.thescizone.com).

CHAPTER 11: MEDICAL COMPLICATIONS OF SCI

Barnett, H., and A. Jousse. "Syringomyelia as Late Sequel to Traumatic Paraplegia and Quadriplegia: Clinical Features," in *Syringomyelia,* H. Barnett, ed. Philadelphia, PA: Saunders, 1973 (pp. 129–152).

Bergstrom, N., M. A. Bennett, and C. E. Carlson. "Clinical Practice Guideline Number 15: Treatment of Pressure Ulcers." Rockville, MD: U.S. Dept. of Health and Human Services, Public Health Service, Agency for Health Care Policy and Research, 1994. AHCPR publication 95–0652.

Falci, S. P., et al. "Surgical Treatment of Posttraumatic Cystic and Tethered Spinal Cords," *Journal of Spinal Cord Medicine,* 22, 1999 (pp. 173–181).

Friedman, A. H., and E. Bullitt. "Dorsal Root Entry Zone Lesions in the Treatment of Pain Following Brachial Plexus Avulsion, Spinal Cord Injury, and Herpes Zoster," *Applied Neurophysiology,* 51 (2–5), 1988 (pp. 164–169).

Goossens, R. H., et al. "Shear Stress Measured on Beds and Wheelchairs," *Scandinavian Journal of Rehabilitation Medicine,* 29, 1997 (pp. 131–136).

Griffin, J. W., et al. "Efficacy of High Voltage Pulsed Current for Healing of Pressure Ulcers in Patients with Spinal Cord Injury," *Physical Therapy,* 716, 1991 (pp. 433–442).

Rees, R. S., et al. "Becaplermin Gel in the Treatment of Pressure

Ulcers in Phase II: A Randomized Double-Blind, Placebo-
Controlled Study," *Wound Repair Regeneration,* 7, 1999
(pp. 141–147).

Schurch, B., W. Wichmann, and A. B. Rossier. "Post-Traumatic
Syringomyelia (Cystic Myelopathy): A Prospective Study of 449
Patients with Spinal Cord Injury," *Journal of Neurology and
Neurosurgical Psychiatry,* 60, 1996 (pp. 61–67).

APPENDIX

Jackson, A. B., et al. "A Demographic Profile of New Traumatic Spinal Cord Injuries: Change and Stability over Thirty Years,"
from *Archives of Physical Medicine and Rehabilitation,* vol. 85,
Nov. 2004 (pp. 1740–1748).

Meade, M., et al. "Race, Employment, and Spinal Cord Injury," from
Archives of Physical Medicine and Rehabilitation, vol. 85, Nov.
2004 (pp. 1782–1792).

Stover, S., J. DeLisa, and G. Whiteneck. *Spinal Cord Injury—Clinical
Outcomes from the Model Systems.* Gaithersburg, MD: Aspen
Publishers, 1995 (pp. 25–52).

Acknowledgments

Although this book was first conceived in 2001, the roots of the project go back to when I was first introduced to the world of rehabilitation medicine during my undergraduate years at the University of Michigan in the mid-1980s. Working on research projects with the late Dr. Gary Davidoff, I was strongly attracted to this field, which encompasses not only the science of rehabilitation but also the psychosocial intricacies of disability. Further support came during medical school at Michigan from Dr. Theodore Cole and Sandra Cole, who allowed me to tag along to their weekly clinics, where they helped disabled individuals manage issues of sexuality.

While at the Rehabilitation Institute of Chicago (RIC) for my rehab residency, I was privileged to know and learn from Dr. Henry Betts, a true leader in the field whose wisdom and passion continue to inspire me. In the early 1990s, after my first-hand experience caring for patients both on the acute spinal cord injury unit at Northwestern Memorial Hospital and on the seventh floor at RIC, I decided upon a career focused on SCI. Mentors like Dr. Betts, Dr. David Chen, and Dr. Elliott Roth were invaluable resources for me during these years, passing on their knowledge and sage advice.

Having fallen in love with New England during teenage summers spent at Harvard Summer School and at Massachusetts General Hospital as a research assistant under Dr. Robert Neer, I jumped at the opportunity to return to Boston and Harvard as the first medical director of the Spinal Cord Injury Program at Spaulding Rehabilitation Hospital, a Harvard Medical School–affiliated institution. While the prospects of developing and managing a clinical program right out of residency were daunting, the wise counsel provided by Dr. Paul Corcoran, then Spaulding's director of Physical Medicine and Rehabilitation, allowed me to proceed with confidence. He also introduced me to the world of disability beyond the hospital setting, including the Boston Center for Independent Living, various local agencies dedicated to assisting those with disability, and social outlets such as wheelchair sports groups.

By interacting directly with dozens of patients and families on a regular basis, I became increasingly aware of the many challenges and accomplishments of those facing disability. Thanks to the incredible team of therapists, nurses, and other support staff I had the pleasure to work with, many individuals who were frightened and hopeless upon entering Spaulding left several months later with a sense of direction and hope. Dr. Walter Frontera, who succeeded Dr. Corcoran, carried on the vision for a comprehensive SCI program and for Harvard's entire Department of PM&R.

While I was at Spaulding my colleague and friend Dr. Julie Silver encouraged me to become involved with the Family Health Guides series as author of this volume. An outstanding physician as well as an accomplished writer and contributor to the series herself, Julie gave me the support and guidance needed to navigate the early hurdles of book writing. Dr. Joel Stein, my direct supervisor, also provided sound advice and enthusiastically backed my involvement with the project from day one.

The biggest boost came when my husband, Saul Wisnia, entered the picture. A gifted writer and editor with several books to his own credit, he became the "in-house" co-author I needed to get the project done. Whether pushing me to write after the kids were asleep or lugging our laptop on assorted vacations and holiday trips to Michigan, he was my co-conspirator all the way. He also was invaluable in helping interview the many patients from Spaulding and my subsequent jobs at Whittier and Fairlawn Rehabilitation Hospitals who graciously shared their time and most personal experiences for this book. Our thanks goes out to all of them, especially Cindy and Ted Purcell, who read every page of the manuscript and let us know what did and didn't work. Saul's bosses at Dana-Farber Cancer Institute, Steve Singer and Paul Hennessy, were supportive in allowing him time to devote to the project, and his colleague Debbie Bradley Ruder went above and beyond with excellent editorial advice and insights.

We had an outstanding literary team at Harvard University Press as the manuscript unfolded over the past five years. Ann Downer-Hazell and Christine Thorsteinsson were superb and compassionate editors, and Vanessa Hayes was there whenever we needed her. Artist Arleen Frasca showed great talent and patience in getting each illustration just right. When the unforeseen circumstances of my mother's battle with cancer complicated the journey, the HUP team gave us the extra time and help we needed to see things through.

I want to thank my family: my father, Dr. Edward Alpert, who inspired my career in medicine from early childhood; my late mother, Agi, for being my number-one cheerleader and advocate; Steve, for being my big brother; Saul's family, for their support and babysitting help; and our children, Jason and Rachel, for (usually) giving Mom and Dad the time and space to write.

Lastly, I would like to express my heartfelt appreciation to all my patients and their families—past, present, and future—for continuing to teach me each day about the power of the human spirit and the ability to persevere over adversity through courage and determination.

Michelle J. Alpert

Index

Abdomen, 25
AbleData, 310
Abortion, 203
Acceptance, 72
Access-Able Travel Source, 311
Access for Disabled Americans, 303
Accommodation, mutual, 166–167
Acute care phase, 24–27
Adaptive baby care equipment, 215–220
Adjustments, 53–56, 73; returning home, 56–61; failure to cope, 61–67; coping strategies, 67–72; by children of disabled parents, 204–207
Adoption, 203–204
Agency for Healthcare Research and Quality, 282
Alcohol, 61–64, 282
Alcoholics Anonymous, 64
Alkaline phosphotase, 276
Alliance for Technology Access, 303
Ambulances, transport by, 24
American Academy of Physical Medicine and Rehabilitation, 304
American Association of Spinal Cord Injury Psychologists and Social Workers, 304
American Congress of Community Supports and Employment Services, 308

Americans with Disabilities Act, 43, 74, 96, 104, 204, 215, 247, 309
American Spinal Cord Injury Association, 304
Anemia, 185, 282
Anger, 41–43, 51, 55, 158, 170, 257–260
Ankle braces, 26
Anticonvulsants, 272, 292–293
Antidepressants, 292
Anxiety, 40–41, 54–55, 66, 101, 141, 147, 210
Apathy, 210
Arms, 4, 13–14, 16–17, 25
Assisted reproductive technologies, 174, 181–182
Autolytic debridement, 283
Autonomic dysreflexia, 106, 144, 176–178, 189–190, 240, 266–269

Baby carriers, 216–217
Backboards, 24
Back braces, 25
Baclofen (lioresal), 65, 272–273
Balancing exercises, 30
Bartels, Elmer, 89–91, 94
Basketball, 103
Bassinets, 215
Bathing, 31, 71
Bed mobility, 27, 30
Bed sores. See Pressure sores
Behavioral plans, 32
Birth control, 133, 145–146

Bladder, 7, 14–17, 23, 26, 30, 40, 141–142, 186–187, 239–240, 242, 268–269, 271–272
Bladder stones, 240
Blood clots, 187
Blood pressure, 106, 144–145, 176, 178, 184, 189, 239, 266–269
Body language, 112
Body weight, 185, 282
Bones, 4–6, 8, 275–277
Boston Center for Independent Living, 90
Bottle wraps, 218–220
Botulinum toxin, 273, 293–294
Bowels, 7, 14–17, 23, 26, 30, 40, 141–142, 185, 240, 242
Braces, 14, 25, 31
Brain, 4–5, 16
Brain injuries, 31–32
Breathing, 24, 31, 239
Breathing tubes, 28, 31
Buck, Frances Marks, 206–207
Buildings, access to, 74, 97
Burnout, caregiver, 157–160

Calcium levels, 239
Canine Companions for Independence, 306
Card holders, adapted, 102
Caregiver burnout, 157–160
Caregiving, 162–165
Carepages.com, 47
Carpal tunnel syndrome, 287
Case managers/coordinators, 32, 51
Catheters, 30, 42, 126, 131, 141–142, 180, 240, 268–269
Cauda equina, 5, 7, 15, 288
Central cord syndrome, 17
Central pain, 288–289
Centre for Independent Living in Toronto, 214
Cervical cord, 5, 7–8, 31
Cervical SCI: C1, 4; C2, 4; C3, 4, 9–11; C4, 4, 9–11; C5, 4, 9–11; C6, 4, 9–11; C7, 4, 9–11, 107; C8, 9–11
Cervical spine, 4–6, 8, 25
Chest, 25

Childbirth, 183, 188–190, 209
Childcare, 160–162
Children of disabled parents, 200–211; impact on, 18–19; infants, 211–221; toddlers, 211–231; teenagers, 231–235
Children with spinal cord injury, 236–238; growing pains, 238–244; at home, 244–255; family reactions, 255–264
Christopher and Dana Reeve Paralysis Resource Center, 305
Cialis (tadalafil), 128
Circulation, 24
Client assistance programs, 80
Clinical depression. See Depression
Clothing, 49–50, 118, 125, 216, 278–279
Codeine, 292
Cognitive retraining, 32
Collapsed lungs, 239
Commission on Accreditation of Rehabilitation Facilities, 75
Commitment, 171–172
Community outings, 32, 38, 55
Complications, medical, 265–295
Condom catheters, 131
Condoms, 146
Confidence, 125
Congenital paralysis, 248–252
Constipation, 185
Coping: need for, 56–61; failure at, 61–67; strategies for, 67–72
Cordotomies, 294
Counseling: substance abuse, 63–64; vocational, 75–78, 81–84
Couples, 18, 147–148; reaction to injury, 148–155; going home, 155–156; role changes, 156–165; making it work, 165–172
Cribs, 215–216, 218
Crutches, 14, 118
CT scans, 25, 285

Dating, 110–122, 253–255
Debridement, 283–284
Deep venous thrombosis, 274–275

Delivery, 188–190, 209
Denial, 36–40, 72, 117, 152–153
Dependence, 71
Depression, 43–45, 63–67, 101, 153–
    155, 157, 159, 210, 291
Diazepam (Valium), 65, 272
Diet, 62, 281–282
Disabled Businesspersons Association,
    309
Disabled Sports USA, 312
Discharge from hospital, 32, 54
Discrimination, 74, 115
Discs, intervertebral, 4, 15
Divorce, 170
Dogs, assistance, 306
Donor sperm, 179
Dorsal root entry zone ablation, 294
Double disability couples, 114
Dressing, 31, 71
Driscoll, Jean, 104
Drugs, 61–64
Dysreflexia. See Autonomic dysreflexia

Eating, 31, 69–70, 118
Education Department, U.S., 214
Education of patient, 29
Ejaculate, 174–175, 177, 180–181
Ejaculation, 126, 131, 134, 174, 176,
    178–179
Elbows, 27
Electroejaculation, 178
Emergency rooms, 24–25
Enemas, 240
Enzymatic debridement, 283
Erectile dysfunction, 128
Erections, 126–132, 174, 176
Erogenous zones, 138
Exercise, 62
Extensor spasms, 271

Family/friends: impact of SCI on, 17–
    20; involvement as caregivers,
    26, 29–31; help from interdisci-
    plinary team, 32–33; and pa-
    tient's reactions, 34–35; help to
    patient in rehabilitation, 45–51;
    and return home, 56, 66; reac-
    tions to children with spinal
    cord injury, 255–264
Family Caregiver Alliance, 306–307
Fatigue, 288, 291
Fear, 148–150
Female fertility, 132, 145, 183–190
Female sexual function, 132–133
Fertility, 132, 145, 173–175, 190–196;
    male, 175–183; female, 183–190
Financial issues, 32, 51, 156–157
Flexibility exercises, 30
Flexor spasms, 271
Flying Wheel Travel, 312
Food and Drug Administration, 177
Foreplay, 139, 141
Friends. See Family/friends
Frustration, 41–43, 55, 114, 149, 152
Functional outcomes, complete spinal
    cord injury, 9–11

Gabapentin, 293
Golf, 104
Grief, 43–45, 150, 257–260
Grooming, 31
Guilt, 59, 150–151, 257–260
Gynecologists, 126, 175

Halo braces, 25, 31
Hands, 13, 27
Hand splints, 118
Helicopters, transport by, 24
Helplessness, 148–150
Hernias, 15
Heterotopic ossification, 239, 275–277
Hip dislocation, 239
Hockenberry, John, 95, 118, 228–229
Home, returning to, 53–56; adjust-
    ments, 56–61; failure to cope,
    61–67; coping strategies, 67–72;
    for couples, 155–156; for chil-
    dren with spinal cord injury,
    244–255
Homemaking, 160–162
Home services, 32–33
Hospitalization, initial, 24–27; help
    from family, 45–51; discharge
    from, 32, 54

Hydrocephalus, 250
Hypertonicity. *See* Spasticity

Ideabook on Adaptive Parenting Aids,
    217
Immobilization hypercalcemia,
    239
Independence, 69, 71
Independent Living Centers, 76–77,
    81, 120, 165, 214
Independent Living Movement, 76, 90,
    96
Individual plans of employment, 79
Infants, of disabled parents, 211–221
Information about patient, 47–48
Insurance, health, 32, 54–55, 76, 128,
    131, 182, 293
Intensive care units, 25–26, 28
Interdisciplinary teams, 29–33
International Professional Surrogate
    Association, 143
Intervertebral discs, 4, 15
Interviews, job, 81–85
Intrauterine devices, 145
Intrauterine insemination, 175, 181–
    182
In vitro fertilization, 175–176, 181–182

Job interviews, 81–85
Joint contraction, 26
Joints, 62, 276–277

Kidney stones, 240
Kirschbaum, Megan, 203, 214–215
Kremetz, Jill, 246, 264

Labor, in pregnancy, 188–190
Leg braces, 31
Legs, 4, 7, 13–14, 16–17, 25
Levitra (vardenafil), 128
Ligaments, 4
Lioresal (Baclofen), 65, 272–273
Lumbar cord, 5, 7, 13–15
Lumbar SCI: L1, 4, 7, 9–11; L2, 4, 7, 9–
    11; L3, 4, 9–11; L4, 4, 9–11; L5,
    4, 9–11

Lumbar spine, 4–6, 13–15
Lungs, 239, 274–275

Male fertility, 175–183
Male sexual function, 126–132
March of Dimes, 214
Massachusetts, 76, 90–91, 181, 210–
    211
Massachusetts Rehabilitation Commis-
    sion, 79, 91
Mass Health, 76
Masturbation, 126, 137–138
Mattresses, 26
Mechanical debridement, 283
Medicaid, 90
Medical complications, 265–295
Memory strategies, 32
Menstruation, 183
Microfiber garments, 49–50
Mobility tasks, 27, 30–31
Morphine, 292
Movie theaters, 113
MRIs, 25, 285, 290
Murderball, 57, 106, 313
Muscles, 4, 14, 16, 25–26, 62
Musculoskeletal pain, 286–288

National Dissemination Center for
    Children with Disabilities, 307–
    308
National Family Caregiver Association,
    165, 307
National Institute on Disability and Re-
    habilitation Research, 214–215,
    299
National Parent-to-Parent Network,
    215, 219
National Resource Center for Parents
    with Disabilities, 214, 311
National Spinal Cord Injury Associa-
    tion, 86, 95, 120, 160, 305
National Wheelchair Basketball Associ-
    ation, 103
National Wheelchair Poolplayers Asso-
    ciation, 312
Neck, 8, 24

Neck collars, 24–25
Nerve roots, 6
Neurological evaluations, 25
Neuropathic pain, 288–289
Neuropsychologists, 32
North American Riding for the Handi-
    capped Association, 312–313
Nurses, 30, 32–33, 51, 126
Nurturing Assistance, 213–214

Obstetricians, 190, 209
Occupational therapists, 1, 16, 26–27,
    31
Office of Heath and Human Services
    (state), 78
Olkin, Rhoda, 115, 203, 229
Olympic Games, 88–89, 104
Online dating, 120–121
Oral sex, 139
Orgasms, 134–137
Osteoporosis, 239
Outpatient therapy, 32, 54
Overnight trips home, 54–55

Pain: kinds of, 285–291; treatment of,
    291–295
Panzarino, Connie, 245
Paralympic Games, 104–106
Paralysis, 57, 72; levels of, 8–15; com-
    pleteness of, 15–17; congenital,
    248–252
Paralyzed Veterans of America, 305–
    306
Paraplegia, 3, 13–15, 57, 64, 286–287,
    301–302
Parentification, 221
Parenting, 200–204; dispelling myths,
    204–208; beginning, 208–211;
    infants/toddlers, 211–221; tod-
    dlers/younger children, 221–
    231; older children/teenagers,
    231–235
Parents, reactions to children with spi-
    nal cord injury, 255–260
Partners, impact on, 18. See also Cou-
    ples

Patient-therapist relationship, 1–2
Pendergrass, Teddy, 95, 118
Penile implants, 131–132
Penile injection therapy, 128–129
Penis, 127–132
Personal care attendants, 71, 74, 76–77,
    80, 90, 97, 113–114, 140–141,
    163, 213
Phosphodiesterase-5 inhibitors, 127–
    128
Physiatrists, 29–30, 175
Physical medicine and rehabilitation
    physicians, 26
Physical therapists, 1, 16, 26–27, 30–31
Plate guards, 69
Pneumonia, 31, 239
Positive attitude, 68–72, 117
Postpartum depression, 210
Preeclampsia, 184
Pregnancy, 132–133, 145, 173–175,
    203; challenges, 183–188; and
    parenting, 208–210
Pressure sores, 39, 277–285
Priapism, 129
Productivity, 73–75, 108–109; getting
    connected, 75–77; back to work,
    77–95; back to school, 95–100;
    back to play, 100–108
Prostitution, 142–144
Proteins, 281–282
Psychogenic erections, 127
Psychogenic lubrication, 133
Psychologists, 32, 41
Puberty, 239, 252–253
Pulmonary embolism, 239, 274–275
Purcell, Cindy, 79–80, 82–85, 99–100,
    161, 196–201, 221
Purcell, Ted, 107, 196–199, 275

Quadraplegia. See Tetraplegia

Range-of-motion exercises, 26
Reactions, 33–36; shock/denial, 36–40;
    anxiety, 40–41; anger, 41–43;
    sadness/grief/depression, 43–
    45

Recovery, patterns of, 17
Recreational therapists, 32, 49 101–102
Rectum, 178
Reeve, Christopher, 118, 305
Reflexogenic erections, 127
Reflexogenic lubrication, 133
Registered nurses, 32
Rehabilitation, 1, 15, 18, 54, 73; in
       trauma centers, 25–27; move to,
       27–29; interdisciplinary teams,
       29–33; reactions during, 33–45;
       for children with spinal cord in-
       jury, 241–244
Rehabilitation Act, 80, 97
Rehabilitation nurses, 30
Relationship issues. See Couples
Resentment, 55, 152, 158, 170
Resources, 303–313
Restaurants, 113, 118
Retrograde ejaculation, 176–177
Role changes, 156–165
Role overload, 157
Roosevelt, Franklin, 87
Roy, Travis, 107–108

Sacral cord, 5, 7, 15
Sacral SCI: S1, 9–11; S2, 9–11; S3, 9–
       11
Sacral spine (sacrum), 4–6, 15
Sadness, 43–45, 55, 66–67, 150, 210
Sammons Preston Rolyan, 310–311
Sandwich holders, adaptive, 70
School: returning to, 73–74, 95–100;
       for children with spinal cord in-
       jury, 245–248, 251, 253
Scoliosis, 239
Self-esteem, 66, 68
Self-pity, 56
Self-stimulation, 126, 137–138
Sexual ability, 7, 14–16, 18, 23, 123–
       126, 163, 313; in men, 126–132;
       in women, 132–133; orgasms,
       134–137; exploration, 137–140;
       and loss of spontaneity, 140–
       142; and prostitution, 142–144;
       and sexual surrogacy, 142–144;
       responsibilities, 144–146; need
       to reinvent, 168–170
Sexual Health Network, 313
Sexually transmitted diseases, 146
Sexual surrogacy, 142–144
Sharp debridement, 283
Shock, 36–40
Shoulders, 27
Siblings, reactions to children with spi-
       nal cord injury, 261–264
Sildenafil (Viagra), 128
Skiing, 104–105
Skin, 26, 30, 185–186, 277–285
Sleep apnea, 239
Smoking, 282
Social Security Administration, 76,
       309–310
Social Security Disability Insurance,
       76, 309
Social workers, 32, 51
Spasticity, 187–188, 269–274
Speech-language pathologists, 31–32
Speech therapists, 27
Sperm, 174–181
Sperm motility, 179–181
Spina bifida, 250
Spinal cord: anatomy of, 4–8; trauma
       to, 7–8
Spinal cord injury: degree of function,
       3; statistics, 3, 299–302; learn-
       ing to live with, 3–4, 23–24; lev-
       els of, 8–15; functional out-
       comes, 9–11; completeness of,
       15–17; impact on family, 17–20;
       initial hospitalization, 24–27;
       rehabilitation, 27–29; interdisci-
       plinary teams, 29–33; reactions
       to, 33–45; help from family/
       friends, 45–51; returning home,
       53–72; and productivity, 73–109;
       and dating, 110–122; and sexual
       ability, 123–146; and couples/re-
       lationship issues, 147–172; and
       fertility/pregnancy, 173–199;

and parenting, 200–235; children with, 236–264; medical complications, 265–295; resources, 303–313
Spinal Cord Injury Information Network, 306
Spine (vertebral column), 4–7
Sports, returning to, 73–74, 100–108
Sports, wheelchair, 57, 100–108, 312–313. *See also individual sports*
Spouses, impact on, 18. *See also Couples*
Steroids, 24, 287
Strengthening exercises, 27, 30–31
Stress, 28, 58, 133, 157, 175, 291
Stretching exercises, 27
"Stuffing," 140
Substance abuse, 61–64
Suicide, 64–65
Sullivan, Sam, 87–89
Supplemental Security Income, 76, 94, 309
Support groups, 38, 51
Suppositories, 42, 141
Surgery, 25, 273–274, 294
Surrogacy, sexual, 142–144
Swallowing, 31
Syringomyelia, 290–291

Tadalafil (Cialis), 128
Teenagers: of disabled parents, 231–235; with spinal cord injury, 252–255
Tennis, 105
Tetraplegia, 3, 8, 12–13, 16–17, 28, 57, 64, 71, 106, 112, 280, 286, 301
Tetra Society, 88
Therapeutic recreation specialists. *See* Recreational therapists
Therapist-patient relationship, 1–2
Thoracic cord, 5, 7, 13
Thoracic SCI: T1, 4, 9–11; T2, 4, 9–11; T3, 4, 9–11; T4, 4, 9–11; T5, 4, 9–11, 106; T6, 4, 9–11, 144, 178,

189, 266; T7, 4, 9–11; T8, 4, 9–11, 266; T9, 4, 9–11, 133; T10, 4, 9–11, 176, 188; T11, 4, 9–11; T12, 4, 9–11, 133
Thoracic spine, 4–6, 13
Through the Looking Glass, 203, 214–215, 217–219, 221, 311
Tizanidine, 272
Toddlers, of disabled parents, 211–231
Toileting, 31
Topiramate, 293
Torso (trunk), 4, 14, 25
Tracheostomies, 28, 31
Transcutaneous electrical nerve stimulation, 292
Transportation, access to, 74
Trauma centers, 24–27
Travel, 107, 311–312
Tumors, 15

United States Quad Rugby Association, 313
Urologists, 126, 175

Vacuum-assisted closure, 284
Vacuum erection devices, 129–130
Vaginal lubrication, 133
Valium (diazepam), 65, 272
Vardenafil (Levitra), 128
Ventilators, 28, 31, 64
Vertebrae, 4, 6–8, 15
Vertebral column (spine), 4–7
Viagra (sildenafil), 128
Vibrators, 176–177
Vibratory stimulation, 176–178
Visceral pain, 289–290
Vitamins, 281–282
Vocational rehabilitation counselors, 75–78, 81–84
Vocational rehabilitation services (state), 78–79, 99

Weight, body, 185, 282
Weight gain, during pregnancy, 185
Well Spouse Association, 307

Wheelchairs, 14, 27, 74, 95, 97, 280,
    287; in rehabilitation, 30–31,
    38–40, 52; at home, 54–55, 69,
    71; while dating, 112–113, 118;
    while parenting, 216–220, 228–
    229
Wheelchair sports, 57, 100–108, 312–
    313

Winners on Wheels, 308
Work, returning to, 73–74, 77–95
Wrist splints, 69
Writing, 31

X-rays, 24, 276, 285

Zupan, Mark, 106